Soaps, bubbles
& SCRUBS

NATURAL PRODUCTS TO MAKE FOR YOUR BODY AND HOME

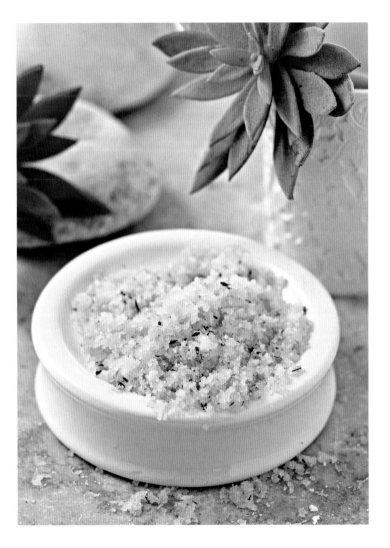

I dedicate this book to my mother. Thank you for passing on all your knowledge and wisdom throughout the years. You have paved the path to my creativity, and I can only hope that I will be as good a mother to my children as you have been to me.

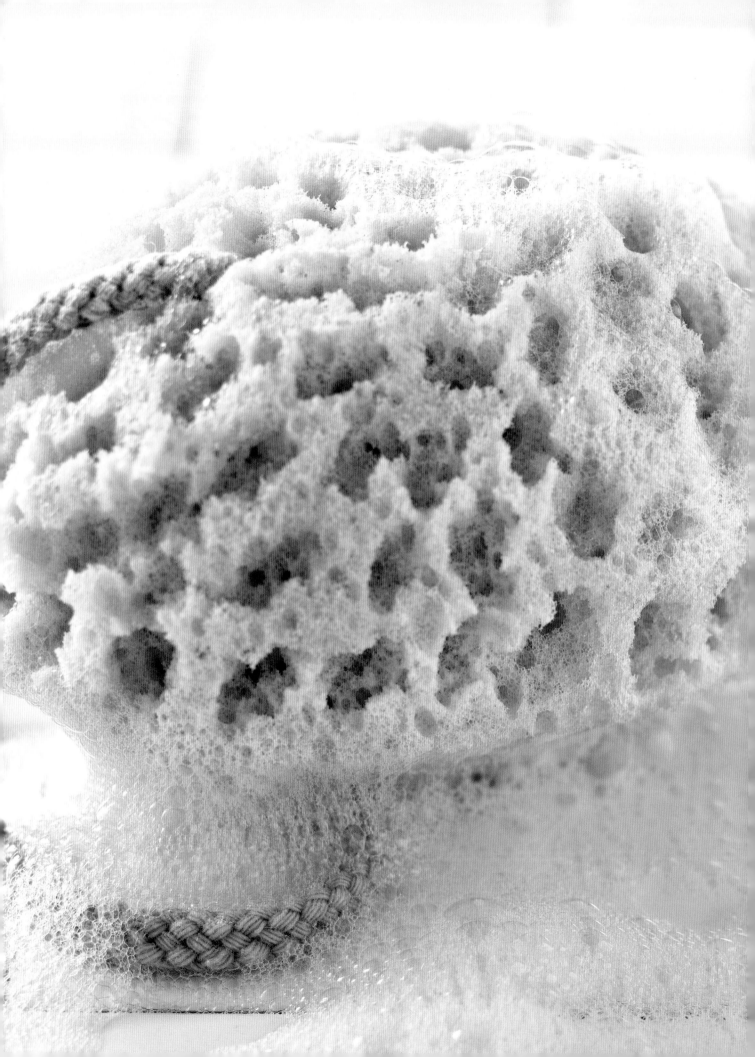

Soaps, bubbles & SCRUBS

NATURAL PRODUCTS TO MAKE FOR YOUR BODY AND HOME

NICOLE SEABROOK

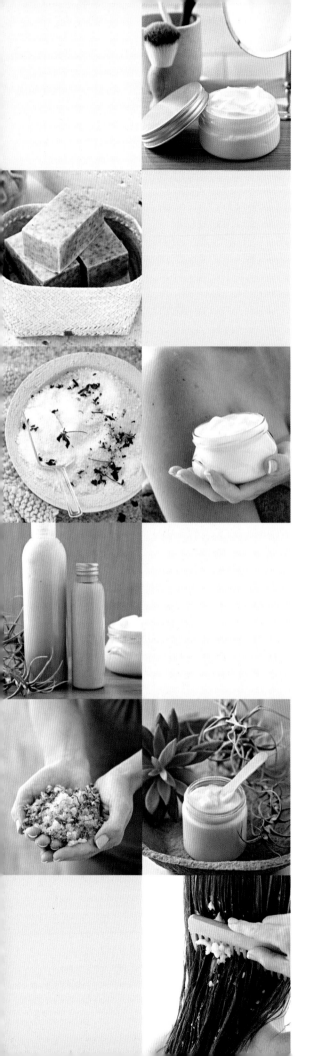

Contents

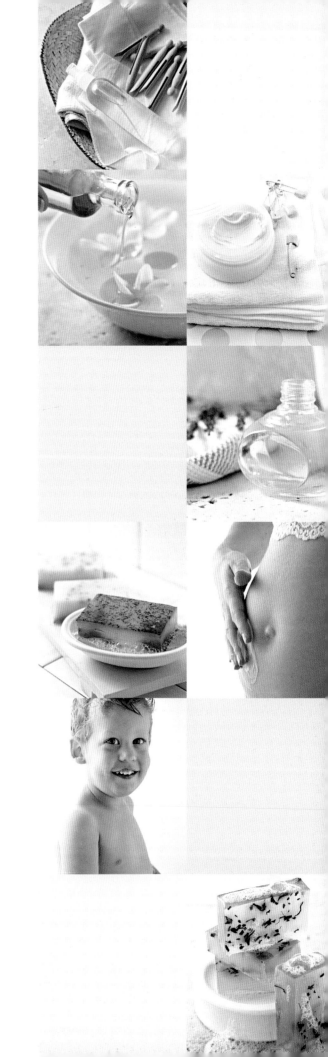

Introduction

I have always loved beauty products. While I was studying Therapeutic Aromatherapy I was introduced to the alchemy of essential oils and their many therapeutic properties. During my studies I attended a workshop on how to make aromatherapy bath and body products and was so inspired that I immediately started experimenting with products for my own use. Eventually, in 2008, I developed my own professional range of products – under the Nature's Way Wellness brand – which I sell to the public as well as to therapists and spas.

There is something so satisfying about creating your very own beauty products from scratch. Every time I try a new recipe I feel like an alchemist mixing and transforming different aromas, waiting for the final product to set, or to turn out a new batch of soap. I can't wait to package the fragrant goodies and send them off to my friends and clients to test and experience.

Over the years I have recommended many remedies to my clients for many reasons, such as a muscle ache bath with Epsom salts and essential oils. Most people don't know what Epsom salts are, where to find them or what quantities to use or what and how much essential oils to use. Through many tests and tweaks I have built up a substantial list of tried-and-tested recipes for a range of situations and ailments.

Years ago, when my mother came across a recipe on how to make soap, I originally thought the concept was silly. Why not just buy soap from the shops – it's only soap after all? The home-made soap turned out to be a great success and it was such a fascinating process that we have never purchased soap again!

Since that time, I have been inspired to create my own natural products and soap, without synthetic fragrances and using only natural essential oils. My clients still rave about the home-made soap and are always giving me new ideas and inspiration to try new recipes and create new blends based on their favourite essential oils. What started off as a few simple ideas has escalated into a whole collection of soap recipes.

Since becoming a mother, I have expanded my products to include a full range for babies. The ingredients in many common baby care products include synthetically fragranced and mineral oils/petrochemicals, which are derivatives of petrol by-products. There are so many natural ingredients that can be transformed into beautiful and eco-friendly products without the use of too many chemicals. I decided to use only the best products for my child. Who wouldn't want to use the best on that gorgeous unspoiled skin?

Making your own soap and home-made spa products from simple household ingredients is fun, creative and cost effective, and they make great gifts.

The recipes in this book have been formulated for the most un-domestic goddess! They are easy to follow and the ingredients are available at most health shops and pharmacies. A lot of the recipes even make use of ingredients that you will probably find in your kitchen.

I have written this book because I would like to share my passion for natural ingredients and fragrant aromatherapy oils combined with the art of creating a craft product that can be utilized and shared, wrapped up as a gift, or just used by yourself! I hope that the simplicity of these recipes will inspire you to create your own products.

NICOLE SEABROOK
www.natureswaywellnes.co.za

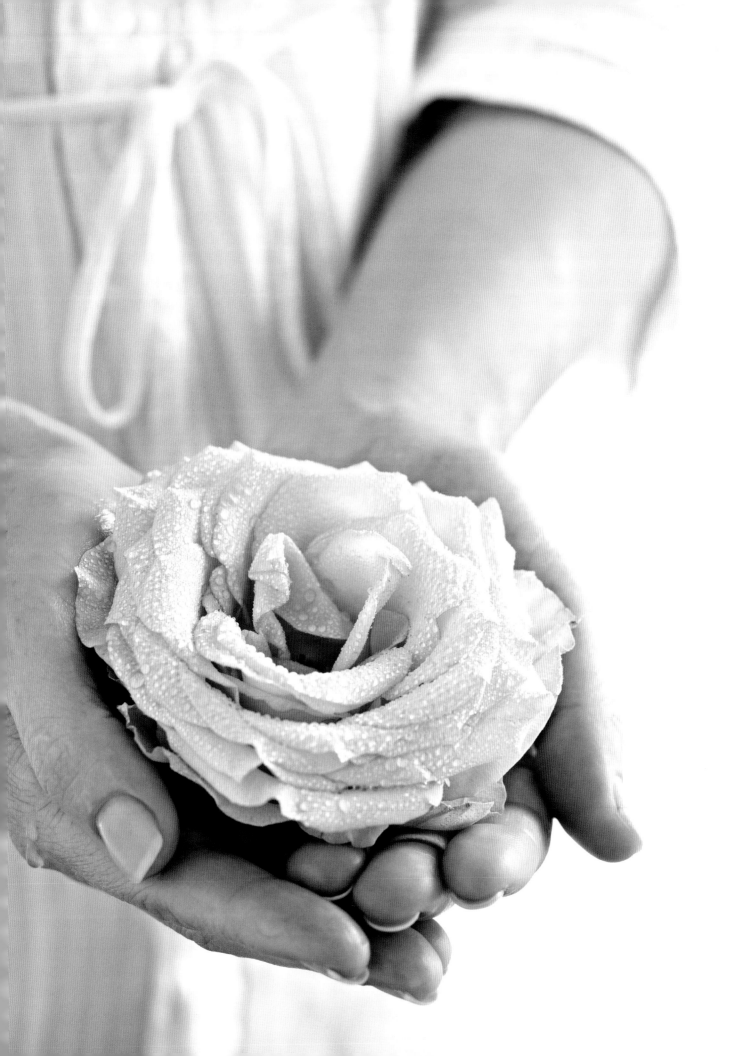

About natural skin care

YOUR SKIN – MORE THAN JUST A BARRIER?

Our skin is our barrier against the outside world – Paracelsus, a renowned physician of the Renaissance who pioneered the use of chemicals and minerals in medicine, called it the royal robe of mankind! This complicated, three-layered organ has many more functions than simply to cover and protect everything inside our bodies.

Healthy, youthful-looking skin has a healthy, natural protective film that is secreted from the glands in the skin itself. This is called the skin's acid mantle. The acid mantle is slightly acidic and has a pH of 4.5–6. It consists mainly of sebum (a secretion from the sebaceous gland) as well as sweat, dead skin cells, waste products and salts. The acidic layer is an unsuitable environment for bacteria, preventing these invaders from entering the body through the skin.

Underneath the epidermis is the dermis layer, which consists of hair follicles, sweat glands, sebaceous glands, blood vessels and nerves. This connective tissue also contains collagen and elastin fibres for support and structure.

The layer underneath the dermis is called the subcutaneous layer or hypodermis, and contains fatty connective tissue for heat insulation and larger blood vessels and nerves.

The skin also plays an important role in temperature regulation. When you get too cool, you get 'goosebumps' when the tiny hairs on the body stand erect and help to trap air and heat, keeping the body warmer. Sweating is the body's response to an increase in temperature – the sweat glands secrete sweat to keep the body cool.

The skin is the largest organ in the human body and is capable of absorbing products, which ultimately get absorbed into the bloodstream. This is great if the beauty products you use on your skin are predominantly natural and contain ingredients that can nourish and revitalize the body, but not always a good thing if the beauty products contain more harmful chemicals than good, natural ingredients.

Natural skin care products help to provide moisture and protection for your skin. Plant-based oils like olive, sweet almond and grapeseed oil, to name a few, have the ability to penetrate the skin and nourish the skin cells with vitamins, minerals and antioxidants, giving you radiant-looking skin.

Natural skin care products do not contain any synthetic fragrances or artificial colours, and only rely on natural aromatic plant extracts, such as essential oils, for their scent. Certain essential oils such as frankincense and lavender can help to rejuvenate the skin by increasing skin cell turnover.

Natural skin care products also make use of natural colours, which have been extracted from plants, minerals and animals.

Here are some examples of natural colouring which may be used in natural skin care products, soap or make up:

Spices: Turmeric (light yellow), paprika (light peach), cinnamon (beige or light brown)

Seeds: Annato colouring from achiote seeds (orange/yellow)

Roots: Alkanet (purple/blue)

Leaves and stems: Henna (dark brown)

Vegetable extracts: Beetroot juice or powder (purple/pink), carrot oil (orange), spinach powder (green)

Algae: Spirulina (green)

Flowers: Essential oil of German chamomile (light blue), saffron (yellow)

Natural compounds such as iron oxides, mica, titanium dioxide: Derived from the earth (brown, black, red, blue, green, white)

Natural colours in skin care are less consistent and stable than artificial colours, and it is for this reason that many natural products tend to be without colour.

We are often fooled by 'natural looking' products, packaged and advertised as containing herbal extracts. They sound natural, but what you don't know is how many other chemicals are lurking in your 'natural botanical' shampoo!

We usually stop to read food labels and ingredients before purchasing groceries, so why not do the same for your beauty products and cosmetics? It is your right as a consumer to know what ingredients your beauty products contain – and even better if you can learn how to create your own natural cosmetics.

All beauty products have an ingredient listing (often in very fine print). If you are thinking of using natural skin care products, there are certain chemical ingredients you may want to avoid:

Petrochemicals

Petrolatum is a chemical by-product of the petroleum industry, and petroleum jelly and aqueous cream are derived from petrolatum. These mineral oils can disrupt the moisture balance in your skin and clog the pores, interfering with your skin's ability to eliminate toxins.

Isopropyl alcohol, ethyl alcohol, ethanol (also derivatives of petrochemicals) are harsh astringents and solvents that can dehydrate your skin. Sodium laureth/lauryl sulphate can cause skin irritations, dandruff and allergic reactions (see also Squeaky clean, page 9).

Propylene glycol (PG), polyethylene glycol (PEG)

Propylene glycol can be made by mixing vegetable glycerine with grain alcohol – both natural products – and used in cosmetics as a humectant (a substance that is used to retain water content) instead of using the usual synthetic chemical mix. PG may cause allergic reactions and skin sensitivity, and may even impair kidney function if used in high concentrations. PEG is used in cosmetics as an emulsifier and penetration enhancer, which could allow other harmful ingredients to be absorbed through your skin.

Synthetic dyes

When listed on a product, synthetic/artificial colours will appear as FD&C (food, drug and cosmetic), followed by a number – such as FD&C Red #3. Artificial colour is often present in eye make-up powders and rouge powder, foundation, lipsticks and lipgloss, etc.. FD&C dye is often derived from coal tar. Synthetic dyes can irritate the skin and have also been found to increase blackhead formation.

Artificial fragrances

Fragrances are one of the top allergens known to trigger asthma attacks and skin irritations. Phthalates (chemicals often found in synthetic fragrances) have been linked to hormone disruption within the body, fertility problems and birth defects. Diethyl phthalate (DEP) is particularly damaging to the male reproductive system and may cause sterility. Most cosmetics don't list phthalates on the label and instead use the term 'fragrance', which is often a chemical mix containing phthalates.

Paraben preservatives

Most commercial beauty products and bath/body products and cosmetics contain chemical preservatives. Parabens (often listed as methylparaben, propylparaben, ethylparaben, isopropylparaben, butylparaben) are examples of chemical preservatives that enhance the shelf life of commercial beauty products and prevent bacterial growth.

Parabens have received some bad press and there is a lot of controversy surrounding them – manufacturers of these chemicals, and the chemical cosmetic industry who use parabens in very small quantities, claim parabens are harmless. Parabens may have the ability to mimic hormones like oestrogen and research has shown that parabens can be linked to cancer. Breast cancer tissue biopsies have revealed a presence of parabens, indicating that these chemical preservatives may not be completely excreted by the body.

Natural cosmetics do not make use of parabens and instead use natural ingredients to preserve their products.

SQUEAKY CLEAN – IS IT REALLY A GOOD THING?

Most commercial cosmetics and beauty products contain chemical foaming agents, such as sodium laureth sulphate (SLES) or sodium lauryl sulphate (SLS). These chemicals are very powerful degreasers and can literally strip the skin of its natural acid mantle. Traditionally SLES and SLS were manufactured for industrial use and they are still widely used today in many of these products, such as car shampoo, harsh cleaning detergents and engine degreasers. These days almost all commercial beauty products that have a foaming action also use them (for example foam bath, shower gel, hand soap, shampoo, face wash, and so on).

Beauty and cosmetic care products and soap should be gentle enough to cleanse the skin, yet maintain its natural acid mantle. Foaming soap agents such as ammonium lauryl sulphate (ALS) and cocamidopropyl betaine (CAPB) – both of which can be derived from coconut oil – seem to be a healthier alternative to SLS and SLES. They are less harsh on the skin and are less likely to cause irritation.

An even better option for sensitive skin is natural homemade olive oil soap, which is made from pure olive oil and beeswax. Generally speaking, natural hand-made soap bars produce fewer soap bubbles with less foaming action, and are therefore more caring and gentle on your skin.

SYNTHETIC FRAGRANCES AND LINKS TO CERTAIN HEALTH CONDITIONS

With nearly all commercial skin care products containing synthetic fragrances, it is not surprising that more and more people are becoming allergic to heavily scented products. Exposure to chemical synthetic fragrances can cause symptoms such as irritation to the ears, nose and throat, as well as headaches and nausea.

If a product is heavily fragranced, it is most likely synthetically produced. Natural aromas/fragrances are derived from essential oils (from plants), whereas synthetically produced fragrances are produced in a laboratory with a variety of chemicals that have been created to simulate the natural aroma.

A large percentage of synthetic fragrances are derived from petrochemicals, which have been known to disrupt the endocrine system, and excessive exposure has also been shown to increase the risk of cancer. Chemicals can be absorbed during pregnancy – via the skin – and high levels of toxic chemicals that have been linked to birth defects are being found in women of childbearing age.

Essential oils do not contain any synthetic chemicals, as they are derived only from a living plant source. Organic essential oils are also free of any pesticide residue that may have been used during the life-cycle of the plant.

The origin of natural cosmetics and the history of soap making

ANCIENT NATURAL COSMETICS AND SKIN CARE PREPARATIONS

It has been claimed that Cleopatra, queen of Egypt, washed with clay and a pumice stone. She also used to bathe in ass's milk and honey, and made use of essential oils for perfume.

Ancient Egyptians – both men and women – used kohl mixed with animal fat to create eyeliner to accentuate their eyes. The dark kohl also helped to lessen the glare of the sun and it was believed that it protected the eyes from disease. The make-up was also applied as a religious ritual to honour their gods.

The bright green colour in ancient make-up was made by crushing malachite, while red make-up was achieved by using red ochre – a natural pigment made from red clay – hydrated iron oxide as well as carmine beetles which, when crushed, produced a deep red colour. Make-up containing these natural pigments is still available today.

Henna, produced from the henna shrub, was also used to colour the skin and hair and to paint and decorate the body. It is still used today.

During the Middle Ages and throughout the Renaissance, women and men used lighteners on their skin (particularly their faces). Having a pale complexion was thought to be aristocratic, as only the upper class did not work and spent most of their days indoors.

In Elizabethan times, a commonly used skin whitener called ceruse was made from white lead. This beauty product was toxic and users often experienced disorders such as hair loss and stomach complaints, and even death could occur if used frequently!

MODERN SKIN CARE AND COSMETICS

Don't think that modern make-up and cosmetics are that safe either. How much lipgloss and lipstick, loaded with petrochemicals and synthetic colour, do you apply during the day? Your lip products could be ending up in your digestive system!

Ingredients present in most lip care preparations contain petrochemicals, such as the mineral oils petrolatum and liquid paraffin. These chemicals tend to make the skin drier and therefore do exactly the opposite to what they are intended to do in the first place.

Foundation that boasts many hours of coverage is bound to cause more breakouts and skin eruptions, while other make-up such as eye shadow and rouge powder containing synthetic FD&C dyes have also been linked to skin irritation.

But there is good news … There is a wide variety of natural and organic make-up on the market that can still keep you looking good – without the harmful chemicals. I love using the Dr. Hauschka® cosmetic range. The products are free of any synthetic colours, artificial fragrances or synthetic preservatives, and only use natural ingredients that have an organic and biodynamic origin.

SOAP MAKING

A soap-like substance has been found in Babylonian clay cylinders dating from as early as 2 800 bce. Historians believe that almost 5 000 years ago, the first soap makers were Babylonians, Mesopotamians, Egyptians, as well as the ancient Greeks and Romans. This raw form of soap was produced by mixing animal fat, oils and salts.

According to ancient Roman legends, soap got its name from Mount Sapo. When animal fat from sacrificial rituals combined with wood ash (alkaline salts) and was washed down the mountain and into the Tiber River, women washing laundry in the river soon realized that the clay soapy substance present on the river banks made their laundry cleaner, with less effort.

This mixture of animal fat and alkaline water (from wood ash and rain water) was the very first primitive soap-like mixture used by humankind.

Ancient soap was not originally intended for bathing and personal hygiene, but was produced for cleaning fabrics, textiles and cooking utensils. This soap-like substance was also used as a base for medicinal ointments and hair pomades (scented ointments).

In earlier times, humans did not bathe frequently. The Greeks and Romans popularized bathing and one of the first Roman baths was built about 312 bce. These public bathing facilities used water from the aqueduct systems. Traditionally, oil was used to anoint the body, and the Romans used implements to 'scrape' off the oil – along with the dirt from the skin. They may also have used sand and pumice stones (which have abrasive properties) to cleanse their bodies.

The volcano, Mount Vesuvius erupted in 79 ce in Pompeii, Italy, revealing an entire soap production factory – including preserved soap bars!

After the fall of the Roman Empire, however, bathing became more infrequent and the lack of cleanliness lead to the plagues of the Middle Ages.

Soap making was perfected in the Middle East, where Arabian chemists used perfumed oils from plant extracts to develop soap recipes. Soap makers guilds were established in the seventh century and soap making recipes became closely guarded secrets. Eventually, however, more varieties of soap became available and basic hair shampoo as well as laundry detergents came into use.

The English began making soap during the twelfth century, using mostly animal fat (tallow). In the fifteenth century France became the soap-making capital of the world and was renowned for using many essential oils and aromatic herbs (especially lavender). By the sixteenth century finer soaps were becoming more available throughout the rest of Europe. Italy, with its abundance of olive groves yielding large amounts of olive oil, first began making soap from vegetable oils instead of animal fat.

For early American settlers the process of making home-made soap was a tiresome chore. Lye water would be made from straining water through wood ash. The lye water was then combined with animal fat and boiled to create soap, which was skimmed off the surface of the water.

In 1791 a French chemist, Nicholas Leblanc, invented a method of making an alkali soda from sodium chloride (NaCl, or common table salt). This chemical process of transforming salt to caustic soda allowed soap to be produced without the time-consuming method of creating lye water from wood ash. Soap production increased and the process became more affordable and less complicated.

During the early eighteenth century in England, fine soap was an item of luxury and was used exclusively by wealthy, upper class citizens. It was only during the Industrial Revolution when raw materials were easily available and the soap tax was finally abolished that soap making became more popular and accessible to all classes. By the end of the nineteenth century most households commonly used soap.

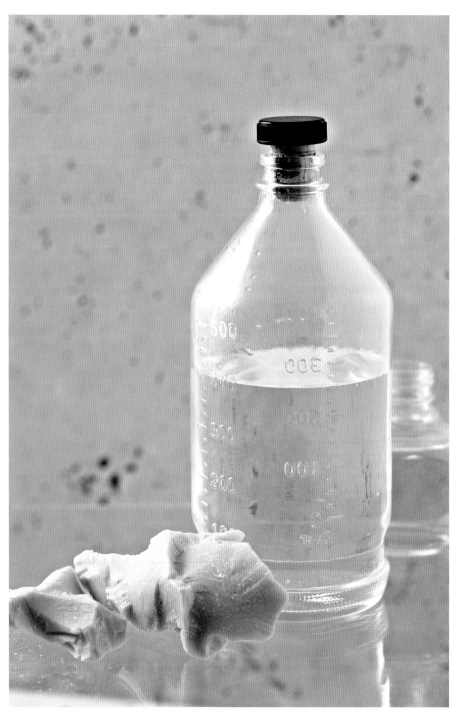

Aromatherapy essential oils

HISTORY AND ORIGIN OF ESSENTIAL OILS – NATURE'S OWN PERFUME

The ancient Egyptians made use of aromatherapy essential oils during embalming rituals. Myrrh and cinnamon were placed in the abdominal cavity during the mummification process to help prevent decomposition, and cedar oil, known for its antibacterial properties, was rubbed onto the skin as a preservative.

Kyphi, an incense made from aromatic plant materials such as myrrh, saffron, juniper and cardamom, and other ingredients like honey and wine, was used by the Egyptians as perfume and offered to the gods. Later, Greek physician Dioscorides made use of kyphi recipes as healing salves and medicinal lotions in his 'materia medica'.

Aromatherapy spread from Egypt, Greece, India and China to all parts of the world, and the use of medicinal herbs and plant extracts is evident in every culture.

Hippocrates, the father of medicine, made use of many plant extracts for healing purposes. He was reputed to use herbal or aromatic fumigations and commonly used herbal extracts for aromatic and medicinal benefit. 'The way to health is to have an aromatic bath and a scented massage every day' – Hippocrates, circa 500 BCE.

Greek physicians and military surgeons were part of the Roman Empire. Galen, who was one of these surgeons and physician to Marcus Aurelius, invented the first 'cold cream' recipe. He made use of herbal poultices and a healing balm enriched with myrrh and olive oil. It was reported that no soldiers died from war wounds during his time served as physician to the army.

During the eleventh century in India, Avicenna invented a very effective way of extracting the essential oils from plants. He used a coiled copper pipe in the distillation process, which allowed for rapid cooling and condensation. Avicenna went on to become a famous physician, philosopher and mathematician. He described over 700 medicines from plants as well as from aromatherapy oils. His work on aromatherapy oils became known as *Perfumes of Arabia* and became widespread across Europe.

The study of plants and humankind has enabled us to make use of plants' healing properties to help create balance and harmony within our bodies. Scientific studies of essential oils have shown positive changes in the brain, affecting the mind as well as the emotions.

In 1928 René-Maurice Gattefossé, a French chemist, coined the term 'aromatherapy'. He was working with lavender oil (used for perfume) in his laboratory, when a small explosion occurred. He accidentally immersed his burnt arm in the container of lavender oil – and began to notice something very interesting … He observed that the wound healed well, and this sparked an interest in investigating the chemical components of this plant extraction.

He soon realized that the plant extracts had many therapeutic effects on the body, and different essential oils contained different chemical compounds, making them a valuable natural healing aid. In 1937 he wrote a book called *Gattefossé's Aromatherapy*, explaining his scientific findings of these precious healing essential oils.

Did you know? Lavender is one of the most popular essential oils in aromatherapy. Dried lavender has been used for centuries, and sachets of the dried plant were kept in linen drawers and cupboards to help keep insects and moths at bay. The Greeks and Romans also bathed in and washed with lavender water, as it was well known for its antiseptic properties and fresh aroma. The Latin word lavare actually means 'to wash', and is presumably the origin of the name lavender.

WHAT IS AROMATHERAPY?

Aromatherapy is the word used to describe the use of aromatherapy essential oils for physical and psychological well-being. Aromatherapy is the art of using essential oils combined with rhythmic, gentle massage.

Aromatherapists make use of essential oils in various ways to help create balance and harmony:

Aromatherapy massage
Compresses (cool compresses for headaches, sunburn, fever; warm compresses to ease backache, abdominal cramps, arthritis)
Applications (like creams and lotions)
Aromatherapy baths
Inhalation (via steaming and vapour mist sprays – useful for sinus infections and sore throats)

WHAT ARE ESSENTIAL OILS?

Essential oils are the concentrated aromatic oils that are extracted from raw plant material. These essential oils are widely used in holistic therapies, like aromatherapy and naturopathy, to help treat and create balance and harmony by easing distress in the physical body.

Essential oils can be extracted from various parts of the plant, for example:

Flowers: jasmine, lavender, neroli, rose
Leaves: rosemary, eucalyptus, basil, peppermint
Wood: rosewood, cedarwood, sandalwood
Seeds: coriander, aniseed
Berries: juniper, allspice
Roots: ginger, vetiver
Peel/fruit: orange, lime, lemon, mandarin
Resin: frankincense, benzoin, myrrh

HOW ARE ESSENTIAL OILS PRODUCED?

There are various ways to obtain essential oils:

Steam distillation method

Steam distillation is the most popular method of extracting essential oils.

Raw plant material – flowers, leaves, wood, bark, roots, seeds, or peel – is placed into water. The water is heated and steam passes through the plant material, vaporizing the volatile compounds. This then flows through a cooled coil, where it condenses back to liquid, which is then collected in the receiving vessel of the distillatory apparatus.

The essential oil has a lower density than the aromatic water and is left floating on the surface. The oil is then separated from the water.

The aromatic water is referred to as a hydrosol or hydrolat. Examples of common floral waters include rose water, lavender and orange blossom water.

Expression method

Most citrus peel oils are expressed mechanically by placing them in a press and squeezing/crushing until the oil is extracted. Large quantities of oil are found in citrus peel, and this makes citrus essential oils more cost effective in comparison to essential oils with a lower yield.

Enfleurage method

This method was used in ancient times before people had access to the modern machinery that we make use of today.

Flowers rich in volatile oils are placed onto ceramic or stone plates that have been coated with a layer of fat (traditionally animal fat or tallow was used, but vegetable fat such as palm oil is also suitable). The aromatic oils permeate the fat as the plant matter decays, with new plant material being added to replace the old. Certain flowers yield more essential oils than others. Tuberose, for example, is replaced after 12–24 hours, jasmine is

replaced every 24 hours and frangipani flowers can be replaced every 48 hours. The process of replacing flowers is completed when the fat mixture is completely saturated by the essential oils. This mixture is called a pomade.

The pomade is dissolved in alcohol and then the alcohol is evaporated, leaving only the essential oil. Essential oil produced in this way is known as an absolute.

Enfleurage is not commonly used today except to produce oil of tuberose, an extremely expensive essential oil only used in the finest perfumes.

Solvent extraction method

A solvent such as hexane or carbon dioxide is used to extract volatile oils from plant matter. This mixture is called a concrete. This method is commonly used for extracting essential oils such as rose, jasmine and ylang ylang.

Ethyl alcohol, a natural alcohol, is used to extract a finer, more concentrated essential oil from the concrete. The alcohol is then removed by evaporation, leaving behind the absolute. Neroli absolute is an example of this method of extraction.

A resinoid is the term used to describe resinous plant matter that has been produced by solvent extraction. Plant resins such as frankincense, myrrh and benzoin are extracted in this way.

Did you know? It takes about 100 kg of lavender to produce approximately 3 kg of lavender essential oil, and 100 kg of rose petals to produce 500 g of rose essential oil.

HOW DOES THE SKIN ABSORB ESSENTIAL OILS?

The skin is permeable to fat-soluble substances and relatively impermeable to water-soluble substances.

Essential oil molecules are so small that when they are applied to the skin (especially within a carrier oil, see page 16) they are able to pass through the epidermis (the outer layer of the skin). Essential oils can also enter the skin through the hair follicles and the sweat glands.

Essential oils are transdermal, which means they can penetrate the layers of the skin to reach the dermis (the bottom layer of the skin), which is rich in blood capillaries. The essential oils can then permeate into the tiny blood capillaries and enter the bloodstream. They are eliminated by the body via the kidneys, liver, skin or the lungs.

THE AROMA-CHEMISTRY OF ESSENTIAL OILS – HOW THE DIFFERENT PROPERTIES OF ESSENTIAL OILS ARE DETERMINED, AND HOW THEY CAN AFFECT THE PHYSICAL BODY

Since essential oils are derived from plant matter, they are often rich in antioxidants, and have anti-bacterial and anti-fungal properties. The plants naturally depend on these properties of the oils to survive and the oils often play a vital part in the plants' immune system and general health. By using these extracts of nature, we too can help boost our immune system and help to strengthen our vitality.

Each essential oil has its own unique aroma, chemical composition and therapeutic properties. Essential oils are highly concentrated plant matter made up of hydrocarbon molecules that can be further broken down into their chemical components.

Different chemical compounds present in essential oils can have very different effects on the body.

Examples of popular essential oils and their use in bath/body care products:

Lavender: sedative; analgesic (pain-relieving) and anti-inflammatory effects

Rosemary: stimulates circulation; useful for easing muscular aches and pains

Neroli (from the flowers of the orange tree): calms the nervous system, helping to calm anxiety and nervous tension and stress-related conditions

Orange: citrus fruity aroma; gentle detoxifier, has a calming effect on the digestive system; uplifting and anti-depressant properties

Lemon: refreshing citrus aroma; useful in treating stiff, tense muscles and joints; disinfectant properties

Lemongrass: uplifting citrus aroma; tonic effect on the body

Ylang ylang: often called poor man's jasmine, which its scent resembles; relaxing and anti-depressant properties; reputed to have a stimulating effect on the body, aphrodisiac

Peppermint: revitalizing and refreshing, improves concentration and focus; cooling and soothing properties

Rose geranium: pleasant, floral, rosy aroma; has a balancing effect on the endocrine (hormonal) system of the body and may help to ease PMS and general stress-related conditions

CAUTION: CONTRA-INDICATIONS OF ESSENTIAL OILS

If you are pregnant or have a serious health condition, consult your aromatherapist before using essential oils.

Certain essential oils may be used during pregnancy to help induce relaxation and relieve stress. The following essential oils are recommended during the first trimester of pregnancy: neroli, sweet orange, petitgrain, mandarin, tea tree.

Lavender essential oil is generally a very safe option. Lavender has a calming and soothing effect on most skin conditions and is safe for use after the first trimester of pregnancy, as well as for babies and children (in very diluted concentrations).

The following essential oils can have a stimulating effect on the hormones of the body and are contra-indicated during pregnancy. It is best to avoid the following essential oils while pregnant:
- clary sage
- cypress
- basil
- coriander
- fennel
- frankincense
- juniper
- marjoram
- thyme
- rosemary
- citronella

Always use a very low concentration of essential oils during pregnancy. As a general guideline, I recommend a dilution of 0.5%. See dilution chart opposite for essential oil dilution with carrier oil.

Certain essential oils may also be skin irritants – avoid use if any sensitization occurs. It is advisable to do a patch test on a sensitive area of skin (like the inside of your wrist).

Allow the product to remain on the skin for a few hours. If no irritation develops, then the blend of essential oils most likely agrees with your skin. Although essential oils are derived from plants, one may still develop sensitivity or an allergic reaction to natural products. If you develop sensitivity wash the area lightly to remove the product, and discontinue use.

DILUTION OF ESSENTIAL OILS WITH CARRIER OILS

1 ml = average of 20 drops of essential oil

Carrier Oil	Essential Oil Dilution		
	2%	1%	0.5%
25 ml	0.5 ml		
50 ml	1.0 ml	0.5 ml	
100 ml	2.0 ml	1.0 ml	0.5 ml
250 ml	5 ml	2.5 ml	1.25 ml

HOW ESSENTIAL OILS CAN AFFECT THE BODY THROUGH THE SENSE OF SMELL

Emotions are also affected by aromatherapy. Did you know that the olfactory centre in the nose creates an instant pathway to the brain?

An aromatic scent can trigger a certain memory. Just think of how the smell of freshly baked bread or a certain cake baking in the oven may remind you of your childhood, or the whiff of a certain perfume instantly transports you to a memory of someone who wears that fragrance. Freshly cut grass may remind you of a certain sport that you used to play, or the smell of coconut suntan lotion can send your mind into a state of relaxation as you are reminded of warm, lazy days on the beach.

The olfactory receptors connect directly to the limbic structure of the brain, which processes emotion (the amygdala) as well as associative learning (the hippocampus), explaining how certain odours or scents can directly trigger emotional connections.

The limbic system (also known as the 'emotional' brain) is responsible for stimulating the release of endorphins (via the pituitary gland), relieving pain and promoting the 'feel good' hormones and balancing the nervous system. This is why essential oils can have such a powerful effect on our mood, sex drive and general well-being.

The various responses of the nervous system depend on the different therapeutic properties of the essential oils used on the body. Certain essential oils have a predominantly stimulating or relaxing/calming effect on the body.

THE CONNECTION BETWEEN YOUR SENSE OF SMELL AND TASTE

The nose is also responsible for most of our taste sensations, whereas the taste buds on the tongue can only distinguish sweet, salty, sour and bitter.

As food or drink enters the mouth, it releases molecules that travel through the nasal passage until they reach the olfactory bulb in the brain, which translates the information as flavour. This is a combination of taste (detected via the taste buds) and smell. The sense of smell plays a vital roll in this process, borne out by the fact that when your nose is blocked and you cannot smell, it is difficult to detect different flavours in food.

Did you know? Newborn babies' sense of smell is conditioned to recognize the smell of their mother's milk. Experiments conducted with mothers who washed one breast after birth have shown that 22 out of 30 babies located the nipple by smell, choosing the unwashed breast.

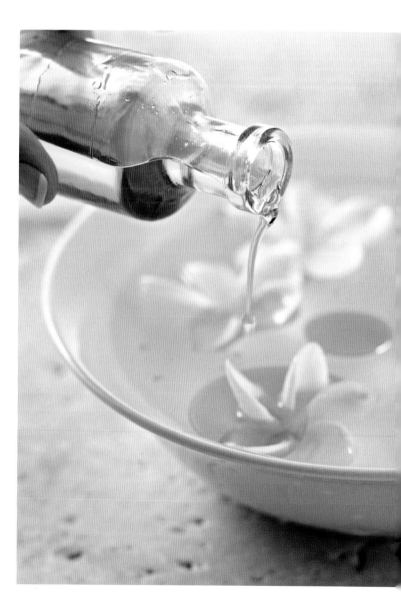

Carrier oils

MINERAL OILS VS PLANT-BASED CARRIER OILS – WHAT IS THE DIFFERENCE?

Mineral oils

These are crude oils that have been extracted from deep within the earth and are considered 'dead oils'. They are also classified as petrochemicals as their origin is generally a by-product of petroleum. The mineral oils available for purchase in supermarkets are generally marketed under petroleum oils and petroleum jelly.

Aqueous cream is made from mineral oils. The base or carrier creams and lotions in this book, however, do not make use of aqueous cream, but rather good quality, therapeutic grade vegetable-based cream that is unscented and suitable for aromatherapy products.

Most baby products contain mineral oils – just look at the colour of the oil (most vegetable oils have a yellowish-golden colour, whereas mineral oils are normally clear).

Mineral oils also have a larger molecular structure than vegetable-based oils and therefore may act as a barrier when applied to the skin.

Commercial baby-care products often use mineral oils within the products to prevent rash (because the mineral oils create a barrier on the skin). I recommend using vegetable-based oil as an alternative because vegetable-based products nourish the skin without creating a barrier, allowing the skin to function optimally yet soothing any skin irritation.

Plant-based carrier oils

Carrier oils – the term used to describe the base oil of the product – are mainly produced from the seeds of plants. The two most popular carrier oils in aromatherapy and Swedish massage are sweet almond oil and grapeseed oil.

Vegetable-based carrier oils are the preferred choice for aromatherapists because of their small molecular structure. This makes them an ideal carrier medium for essential oils, thus enabling the essential oils to penetrate the skin. Essential oils are used to add therapeutic value to the blend of oils used in massage therapy. In order for the essential oils to be absorbed into the skin, vegetable-based carrier oils are used (the molecules of essential oils are suspended within the vegetable carrier oils, making it easier for the blood capillaries to absorb them).

Natural skin care and body products are comprised mainly of vegetable oils.

In soap making you also add vegetable-based oils to the recipes to enrich and enhance the quality of the soap.

This is referred to as 'superfatting'. By adding up to 10% extra oil to the recipe you can enrich the properties of your soap bar.

Some examples of vegetable oils that can be added to soap and aromatherapy skin care products:

Sweet almond oil: Suitable for aromatherapy products and for use in a massage oil blend. Sweet almond oil has skin nourishing properties and is often the preferred choice for aromatherapy massage oil, as it has a good 'slip' and is often used as a carrier oil.

Grapeseed oil: Also ideal for aromatherapy massage as a carrier oil. It has a very thin viscosity and is 'thinner' than sweet almond oil. Grapeseed oil is ideal for oily skin conditions because it has slightly astringent properties.

Olive oil: Thick, viscous oil that is often used in soap making. Excellent healing properties for dry, chapped skin.

Coconut oil: Very thick, semi-solid oil. This oil is used in soap making and is also a popular choice for hair conditioners and skin treatments.

Palm oil: When used in soap, it produces a hard soap bar. This oil is also rich in vitamin E and phytosterols. The rich content of saturated and mono-unsaturated fatty acids makes this oil a popular choice for soap making.

Castor oil: Rich in ricinoleic acid. Castor oil is mostly used in cosmetics and skin care for its wound healing and anti-inflammatory properties. It calms skin infections and relieves itching.

Sunflower oil: Contains gamma linoleic acid (an omega-6 fatty acid), which helps to condition dry, scaly skin. Useful for dry-skin conditions such as eczema and psoriasis. Its anti-inflammatory properties also make this oil a popular choice for massaging aching joints, while easing rheumatic conditions.

Rose hip oil: Extracted from the seeds of rose hips (fruit of a rose). It is rich in omega-3 and omega-6 essential fatty acids and beta-carotene. Rose hip oil is not only useful for maintaining healthy skin, it also increases skin cell turnover, helping to repair skin as well as increase suppleness and elasticity.

Carrot oil: Rich in antioxidants and beta-carotene as well as vitamins B, C, D and E. Carrot oil helps to revitalize and rejuvenate the skin and is often added to cosmetic products to reduce signs of aging.

Jojoba oil: This is actually a wax, not an oil! Jojoba oil is most often used in skin care products due to its emollient properties, which keep the skin supple and hydrated. Jojoba oil closely mimics sebum (natural oils present in the skin), and has both moisturizing and balancing properties on the skin.

Neem oil: Has anti-bacterial, anti-viral, antiseptic and anti-fungal properties. This oil is extracted from the fruit and seeds of the neem tree, which is native to India.

Argan oil: Originates from Morocco. This fine oil is extracted from the fruit of the argan tree, and is commonly used in skin and hair care preparations for its nourishing properties. It is rich in saponins and anti-oxidants, and its high level of vitamin E can also help to relieve itchy skin and calm redness and irritation.

CARRIER BASE PRODUCTS

I mainly use a variety of pre-made carrier base products (produced by a company called Saloncare). The products are made from plant/vegetable oils and contain no mineral oils or parabens. They are also fragrance and colorant free.

Creating your own aromatherapy skin care products is so quick and easy when using pre-made base creams. All that is required is the addition of essential oils, while some recipes are enriched with other carrier oils, such as olive or grapeseed oil.

Saloncare professional products are used by medical practitioners (like homeopaths – who use the base creams in their homeopathic preparations), as well as trained therapists (who use the base products to formulate their own aromatherapy spa products). These base products are available from Saloncare (in bulk), and are also available in smaller quantities from Nature's Way Wellness (single units of 500 g). See contact details on page 151.

These pre-made cream bases vary in viscosity and thickness and are available in the following products:

Carrier lotion: very thin carrier milk, used for bath milk and body lotion

Carrier cream base: used for light body lotion and scrubs, face cream, hand cream

Thickened carrier cream: a very thick cream base, used for body butter and body and facial care products requiring a very nourishing base cream

Carrier gel: water-based gel, used in products that require a cooling effect on the skin

Exfoliant gel: water-based gel with exfoliating wax beads and apricot kernels, used in exfoliating scrub products

Bath milk base

THIS HAND-MADE CREAM RECIPE HAS QUITE A THIN CONSISTENCY AND CAN BE USED AS A REPLACEMENT FOR CARRIER LOTION IN THE AROMATHERAPY RECIPES IN THIS BOOK. THIS RECIPE CONTAINS NO PRESERVATIVES AND HAS TO BE USED WITHIN 4 WEEKS.

MAKES APPROXIMATELY 350 ML

20 g finely chopped or grated beeswax
120 ml distilled water or hydrosol
250 ml sweet almond oil
120 ml witch hazel solution

1. Place the beeswax and water in a saucepan and heat gently until the beeswax has melted. Note that the beeswax will float on top of the water and will not mix with the water. Remove the saucepan from the heat as soon as the beeswax has melted.
2. In another saucepan, heat the sweet almond oil and witch hazel together until warm, but not too hot.
3. Switch on the food processer (on a low setting) and add the beeswax/water mixture. Blend for about 1 minute.
4. Very slowly (with the food processer running), add the warm oil/witch hazel mixture and blend for another minute until it thickens slightly.

Carrier cream base

THIS HAND-MADE CARRIER CREAM RECIPE IS SLIGHTLY THICKER THAN THE BATH MILK CARRIER LOTION RECIPE
AND IS IDEAL AS A SUBSTITUTE FOR ANY AROMATHERAPY RECIPE THAT REQUIRES CARRIER CREAM BASE.
THIS CARRIER CREAM CONTAINS COCONUT OIL, WHICH HELPS TO CREATE A THICKER VISCOSITY. THE RECIPE
CONTAINS NO PRESERVATIVES AND THE CARRIER CREAM HAS A SHELF LIFE OF 4 WEEKS.

MAKES APPROXIMATELY 350 ML

24 g finely chopped or grated beeswax
80 ml distilled water or hydrosol
60 ml coconut oil
250 ml sweet almond oil
100 ml witch hazel solution

1. Place the beeswax and water in a saucepan and heat gently until the beeswax has melted. Note that the beeswax will float on top of the water and will not mix with the water. Remove the saucepan from the heat as soon as the beeswax has melted.
2. In another saucepan, heat the coconut oil, almond oil and witch hazel together until warm, but not too hot.
3. Switch on the food processer (on a low setting) and add the beeswax/water mixture. Blend for about 1 minute.
4. Very slowly (with the food processer running), add the warm oil/witch hazel mixture and blend for another minute until it thickens.

Hand-made body butter

THIS RECIPE CONTAINS ROSE WATER AND COCOA BUTTER – WHICH PRODUCES A THICK, NOURISHING CREAM BASE THAT
CAN BE USED AS A SUBSTITUTE FOR ANY AROMATHERAPY RECIPE IN THIS BOOK THAT REQUIRES 'THICKENED CARRIER CREAM'
AS A BASE CREAM. THIS HAND-MADE BODY BUTTER CONTAINS NO PRESERVATIVES AND HAS A SHELF LIFE OF 4 WEEKS.

MAKES APPROXIMATELY 350 ML

24 g finely chopped or grated beeswax
120 ml rose water and witch hazel
  solution
60 ml coconut oil
250 ml sweet almond oil
40 g cocoa butter
20 g soya wax
5 ml vitamin E oil

1. Place the beeswax and rose water/witch hazel solution in a saucepan and heat gently until the beeswax has melted. Note that the beeswax will float on top of the water and will not mix with the rosewater/witch hazel solution. Remove the saucepan from the heat as soon as the beeswax has melted.
2. In another saucepan, heat the coconut oil, sweet almond oil, cocoa butter and soya wax together until warm. The oils should be melted and the mixture should be warm, but not too hot.
3. Switch on the food processer (on a low setting) and add the beeswax/rose water mixture and blend for about 1 minute.
4. Very slowly (with the food processer running), add the warm oil mixture and blend for another minute until it thickens. Stir in the vitamin E oil.
5. The mixture will thicken more as it cools.

> *Tip:* Use vitamin E capsules (available from your health shop or pharmacy) to boost your skin with antioxidants.
> Vitamin E oil is also useful to add into your creams, as it is a natural preservative. Simply snip the capsules
> open with cleaned and sterilized scissors and add the oil to your favourite cream recipe.

Carrier cream base

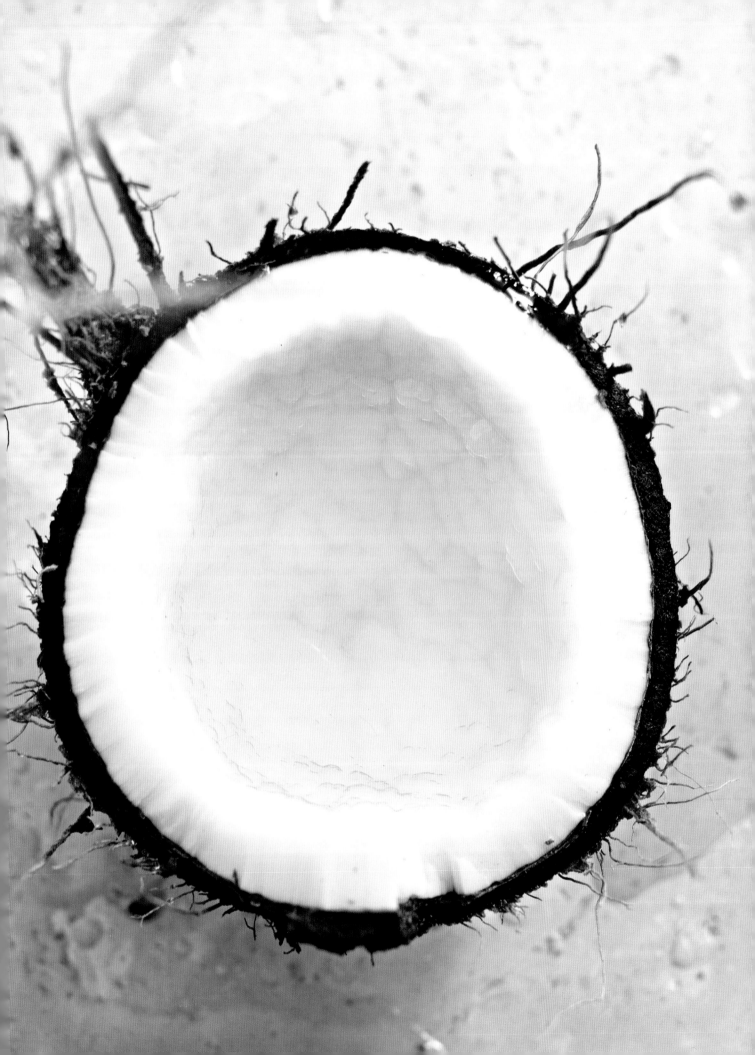

Equipment

Soap making requires minimal financial investment because you will probably find most of the equipment needed in your kitchen, such as measuring cups, saucepans and dischcloths. I like to use a separate two-plate stove for all my soap-making and aromatherapy products, but you can use your kitchen stove too if preferred.

I keep all my plastic soap-making and aromatherapy equipment separate from my kitchen equipment because the essential oils may penetrate the plastic and leave a slight aroma that could permeate food items if the same containers are used. Stainless steel equipment, however, will not absorb aromas and can be used again for preparing foods, etc., but just be sure to wash well after using!

It is important to sterilize all your equipment before use to ensures that the items are clean and sterile. Simply soak the items in boiling water for a couple of minutes and then dry thoroughly using a clean cloth. Remember to sterilize your storage containers and bottles for your products too.

It is advisable to use stainless steel saucepans instead of aluminium when making and melting soap. Aluminium can react with the lye (caustic ingredients) in soap and, when heated, small amounts of aluminium can leach into your products or soap.

Here is a list of items that you will need to get started to make your own soap and natural skin care products:

AROMATHERAPY SKIN CARE AND BATH PRODUCT EQUIPMENT:
- Heavy-duty plastic or glass mixing bowls
- Stainless steel teaspoons/tablespoons for mixing
- Stainless steel measuring cups and spoons
- Large whisk
- Spatula
- Stainless steel saucepans
- Small whisk
- Glass or heavy-duty plastic jug
- Table tennis balls (for making bath fizz balls)
- 2 x dishcloths
- Dried herbs, tea or spices/natural colour for soap
- Essential oils
- Food processer (if you want to make your own carrier creams, lotions and body butter)
- Newspapers (to protect work surfaces)
- Paper towel (to wipe up any spills and also to protect work surfaces)
- Digital scale
- Plastic or glass containers for storing your products

GLYCERINE SOAP-MAKING EQUIPMENT:
- Stainless steel saucepan
- Stainless steel spoon
- Digital scale
- Soap moulds
- 2 x dishcloths
- Dried herbs, tea or spices/natural colour for soap
- Essential oils

COLD-PROCESSED SOAP-MAKING EQUIPMENT:
- 2 x 5-litre plastic buckets
- Digital scale
- Wax paper
- Protective eyewear
- Rubber gloves
- Dust mask
- 2 x dishcloths
- Plastic container/soap mould measuring 18 x 20 x 5 cm deep (this should be sprayed lightly with non-stick baking spray, or greased with coconut oil or white margarine, and lined at the bottom with cellophane paper)
- Long-handled stainless steel spoon (for mixing sodium hydroxide into water)
- Large stainless steel saucepan
- Hand-held stick blender
- Stainless steel whisk
- Plastic spatula
- Dried herbs, tea or spices/natural colour for soap
- Essential oils

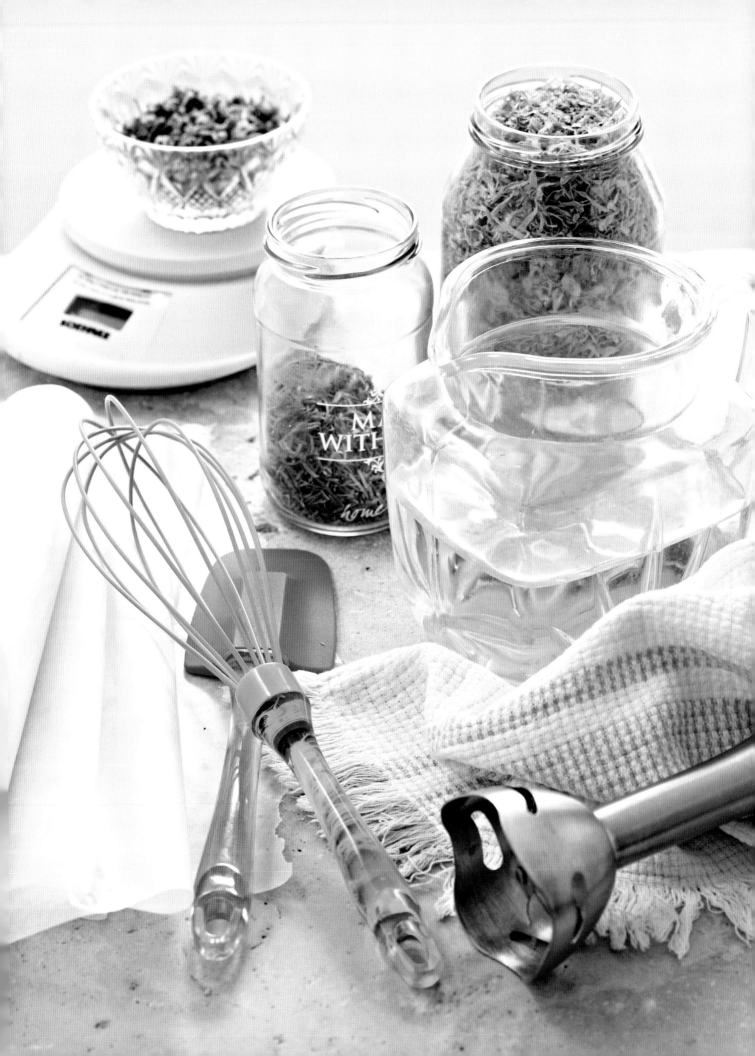

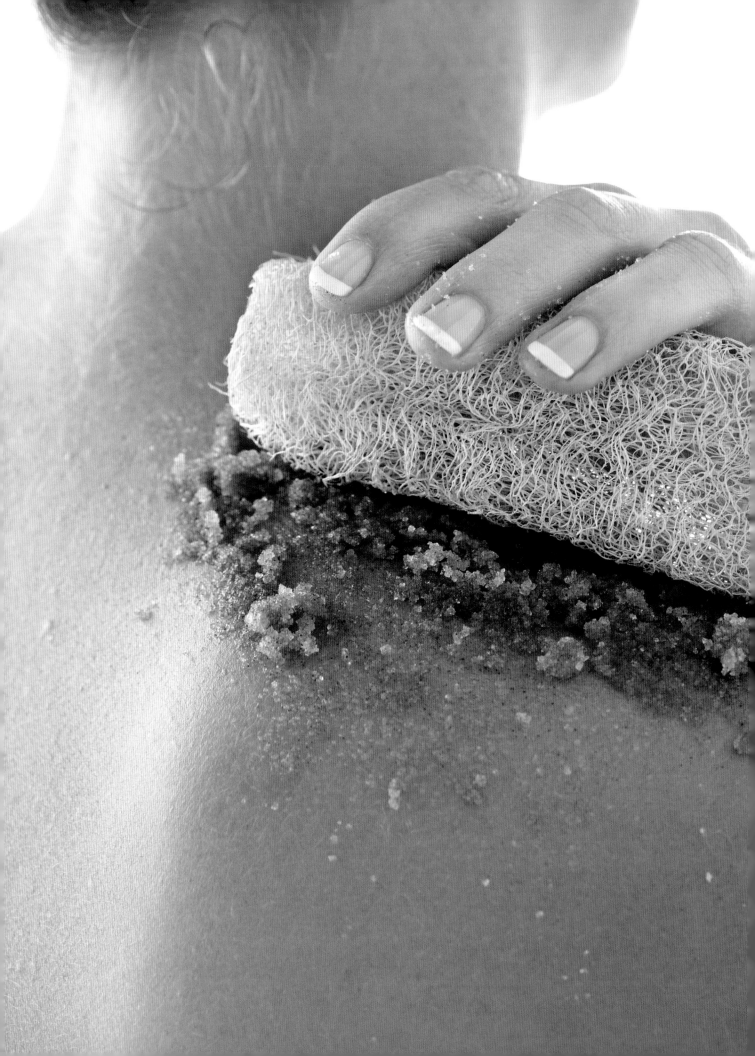

Products for the body

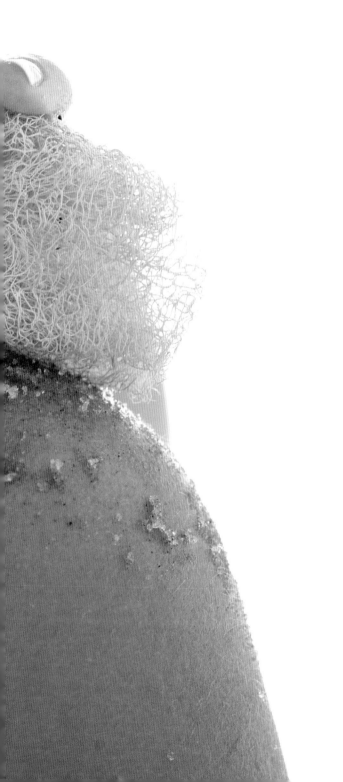

Body scrubs

A BUILD-UP OF DEAD SKIN CELLS CAN LEAVE YOUR SKIN LOOKING DULL. RENEW YOUR SKIN, NATURALLY, WITH THESE SIMPLE BODY SCRUB RECIPES TO INVIGORATE AND KEEP YOUR SKIN LOOKING SUPPLE AND SMOOTH.

Sugar and spice shea butter body polish scrub

THIS BODY POLISH SCRUB WILL LEAVE YOUR SKIN FEELING DELICIOUSLY SOFT AND SMOOTH – SUGAR, SPICE AND ALL THINGS NICE!

MAKES 250 ML

15 ml shea butter
250 ml sugar
15 ml coconut oil
25 ml grapeseed oil
5 ml ground cinnamon
10 drops jasmine essential oil
5 drops sweet orange essential oil
3 drops lemongrass essential oil
7 drops ginger essential oil

1. Mix the shea butter and sugar together and add the coconut oil, grapeseed oil and cinnamon. Stir until the spice and oils are mixed through.
2. Add the essential oils and mix well.
3. Spoon into a sterilized glass jar or plastic tub.

How do I use the scrub? Stand in the shower or on a bathroom mat. Moisten the skin with water, and then apply the scrub onto the skin using circular movements. Do not stand directly under the shower whilst scrubbing as the water will dilute the scrub. Rinse off in the shower. Your skin will feel soft, smooth and polished! This preservative-free product will last up to two months, but the aroma may fade slightly and the oils may start to deteriorate as time goes by.

Exfoliating rosemary and salt body scrub

CLEAN, FRESH AND STIMULATING FOR CIRCULATION, THE ROSEMARY AND THE SALT ALSO HELP TO REMOVE EXCESS DRY SKIN. I PREFER TO USE MEDIUM-GRADE SALT AS THE COARSE SEA SALT IS A BIT TOO ROUGH FOR A BODY SCRUB.

MAKES 250 ML

250 ml medium-grade salt
50 ml sweet almond oil
5 ml dried rosemary
10 drops lavender essential oil
6 drops rosemary essential oil

1. Mix the salt, almond oil and rosemary together in a bowl. Stir in the essential oils.
2. Spoon into a sterilized glass jar or plastic container.

How do I use the scrub? Stand in the shower or on a bathroom mat. Apply to dry skin (moistened with a little water from the shower), using gentle scrubbing movements. Rinse off in the shower.

Citrus, olive and mint body scrub

MAKES 250 ML

250 ml medium-grade salt
50 ml olive oil
grated zest of 1 lemon
5 ml dried mint
5 drops lemongrass essential oil
8 drops lemon essential oil
8 drops sweet orange essential oil
4 drops peppermint essential oil

1. Mix all the ingredients together in a bowl and store in a sterilized, sealed container.

How do I use the scrub? Stand in the shower or on a bathroom mat. Apply to dry skin (moistened with a little water from the shower), using gentle scrubbing movements. Rinse off in the shower. Your skin will feel soft, smooth and polished!

Exfoliating rosemary and salt body scrub

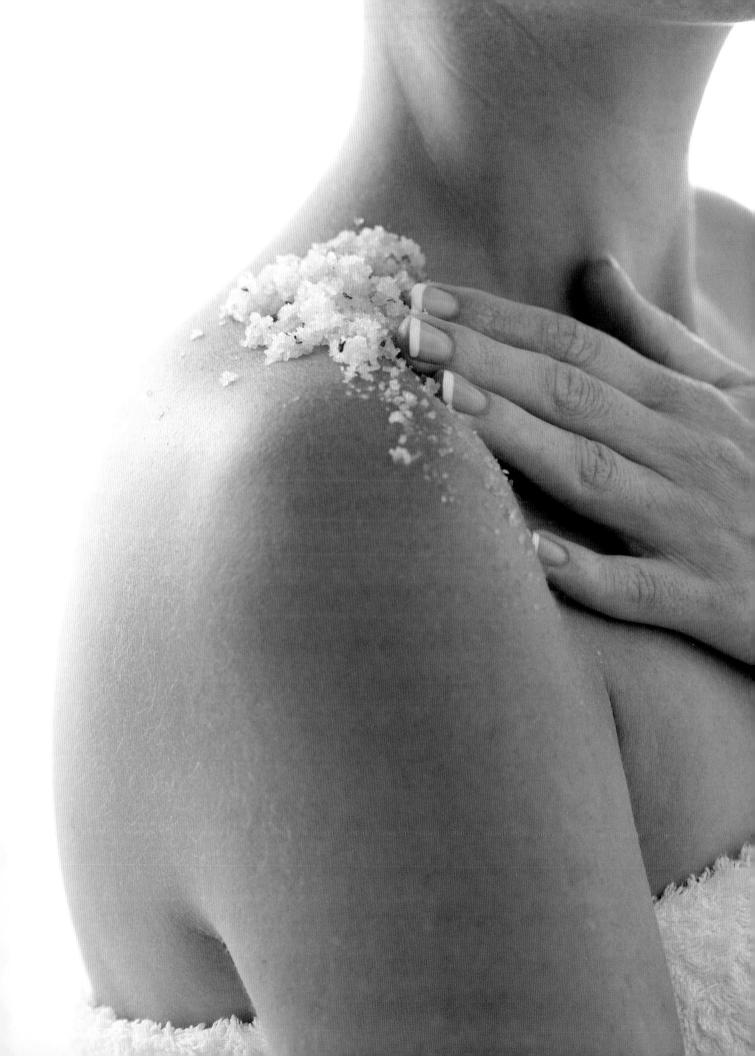

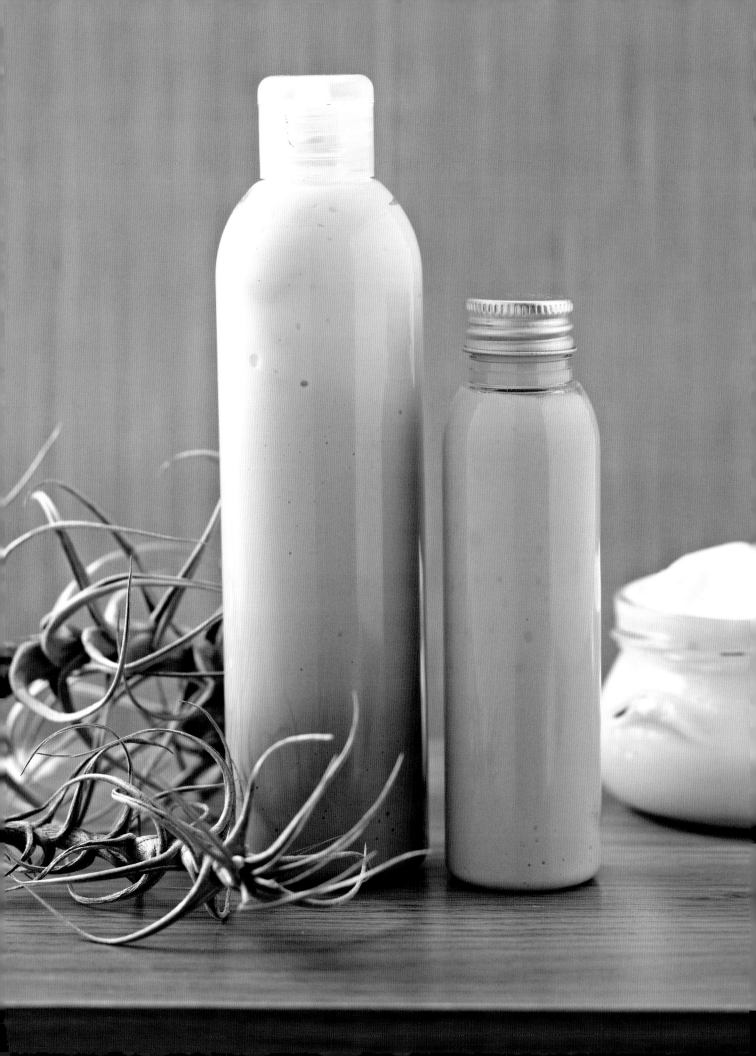

Body lotions

THIS FORMULATION USES PRE-MADE CARRIER LOTION AND CREAM. I PREFER TO MIX THE CARRIER LOTION AND CREAM TOGETHER TO GIVE THE BODY LOTION A LIGHT CONSISTENCY THAT IS SUITABLE FOR NORMAL SKIN OR SKIN THAT IS NOT TOO DRY. BODY LOTION AND NOT BODY BUTTER IS THE PREFERRED CHOICE IN SUMMER, AS THE PRODUCT FEELS LIGHTER ON THE SKIN AND IS VERY EASILY ABSORBED.

African summer body lotion

THINK GORGEOUS AFRICAN SUNSETS, ROOIBOS TEA EXTRACT AND FRESH CITRUS NOTES. THIS BLEND IS PERFECT FOR HOT SUMMER LAZY DAYS.

MAKES 250 ML

5 ml rooibos extract powder
125 ml carrier lotion
100 ml carrier cream
5 ml sweet almond oil
10 drops lemon verbena essential oil
3 drops lemongrass essential oil
12 drops mandarin essential oil

1. Mix the rooibos extract with 5 ml (1 teaspoon) of the carrier lotion and mix well until dissolved. Add the remaining carrier lotion and mix together, then add the carrier cream and sweet almond oil, and mix well.
2. Add the essential oils and mix well.
3. Spoon the mixture into a clear plastic bag and tie in a knot. Snip off one corner of the plastic bag and carefully pipe the mixture into a sterilized plastic container with a pump dispenser.

Sweet dreams body lotion

GENTLY SCENTED WITH LAVENDER AND CITRUS NOTES, THIS BLEND OF CALMING ESSENTIAL OILS MAKES THIS BODY LOTION PERFECT FOR BEFORE BEDTIME. SWEET DREAMS …

MAKES 250 ML

125 ml carrier lotion
100 ml carrier cream
5 ml sweet almond oil
10 drops mandarin essential oil
5 drops neroli essential oil
12 drops lavender essential oil

1. Mix the carrier lotion, carrier cream and sweet almond oil together until well combined.
2. Add the essential oils and mix well.
3. Spoon the mixture into a clear plastic bag and tie in a knot. Snip off one corner of the plastic bag and carefully pipe the mixture into a sterilized plastic container with a pump dispenser.

African summer body lotion

Body butters

THE RECIPES FOR BODY BUTTER ARE FOR A THICK, HEAVY-BASED CREAM – IT'S GREAT FOR NOURISHING THE SKIN AND WILL PROVIDE EXCELLENT PROTECTION IN VERY DRY WEATHER CONDITIONS AS WELL AS HARSH WINTERS. THE ADDED OLIVE OIL HELPS TO MAKE THIS BODY BUTTER EVEN MORE LUXURIOUS. THE SHELF LIFE OF THESE PRODUCTS IS ABOUT 24 MONTHS.

Rejuvenating body butter

ESSENTIAL OILS OF FRANKINCENSE AND JASMINE HAVE REJUVENATING PROPERTIES, INCREASING PRODUCTION OF NEW SKIN CELLS. SWEET ORANGE OIL CAN HELP TO IMPROVE SKIN TONE AND CIRCULATION, AND THE ADDITION OF OLIVE OIL PROVIDES NOURISHMENT FOR DRY SKIN.

MAKES 250 ML

250 ml thickened carrier cream
25 ml extra virgin olive oil
5 drops frankincense essential oil
7 drops jasmine essential oil
12 drops sweet orange essential oil

1. Mix the carrier cream and olive oil together with a small whisk. Whisk carefully until the mixture comes together and then stir in the essential oils. Mix well until all the essential oils have been incorporated into the mixture.
2. Spoon the mixture into a sterilized glass container or plastic tub.

Relaxing body butter

THE MOST POPULAR BLEND – EVERYONE LOVES THIS FRESH, FLORAL, SPICY AROMA! THE ESSENTIAL OILS OF ROSE GERANIUM, GINGER AND ROSEWOOD CAN BE SOOTHING, WARMING AND RELAXING FOR THE MUSCLES, AND ARE REPUTED TO BE A GOOD TONIC FOR THE BODY.

MAKES 250 ML

250 ml thickened carrier cream
25 ml extra virgin olive oil
12 drops rose geranium essential oil
6 drops ginger essential oil
8 drops rosewood essential oil

1. Mix the carrier cream and olive oil together with a small whisk. Whisk carefully until the mixture comes together and then stir in the essential oils. Mix well until all the essential oils have been incorporated into the mixture.
2. Spoon the mixture into a sterilized glass container or plastic tub.

Relaxing body butter

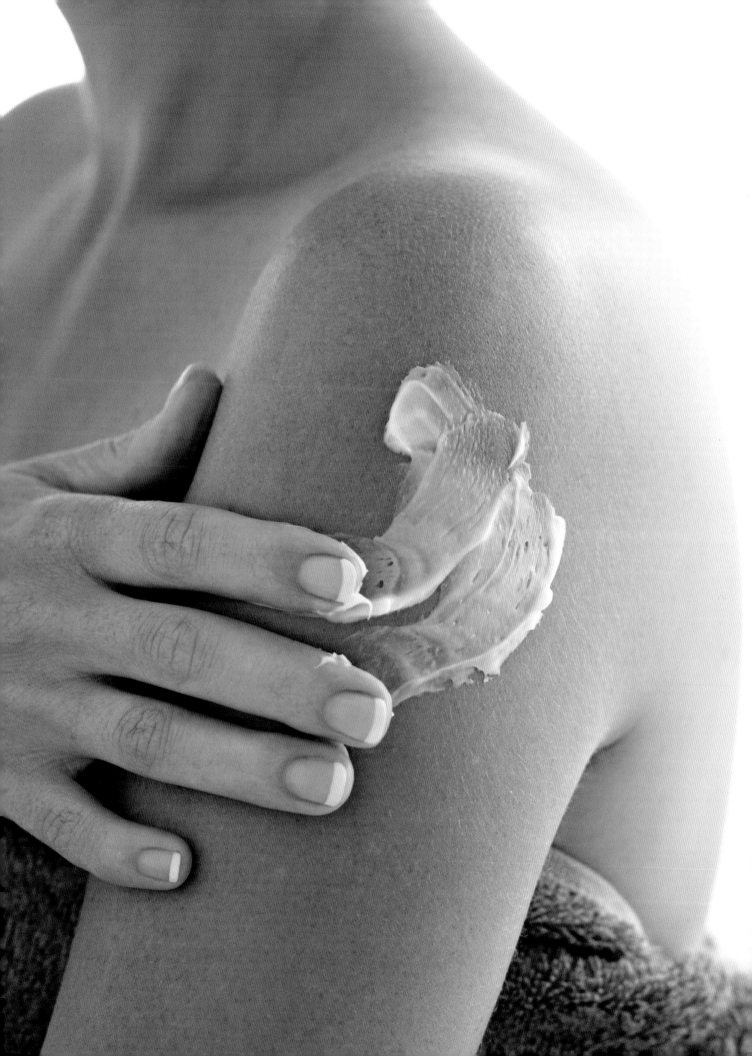

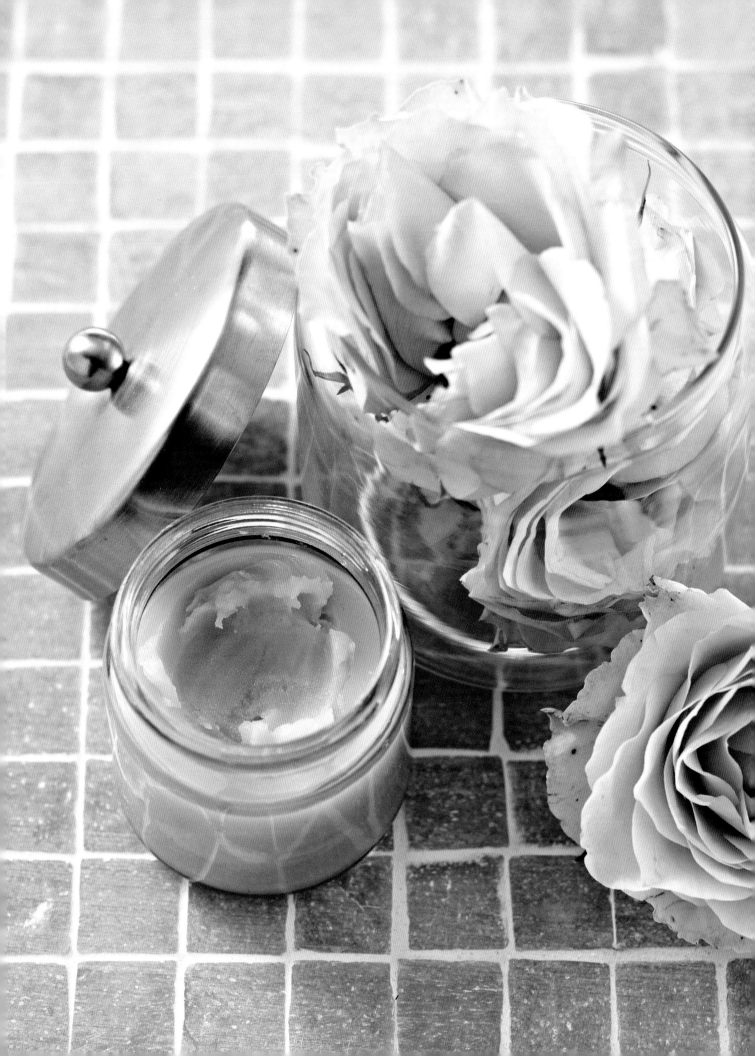

Massage balms

MASSAGE BALM IS EASIER TO TRAVEL WITH THAN OIL (IT WON'T LEAK LIKE OIL SOMETIMES DOES) AND STILL GIVES ENOUGH SLIP, BUT LEAVES THE SKIN LESS GREASY. IT IS ALSO GREAT FOR VERY DRY OR FLAKY SKIN, AS WELL AS ON THE FEET AND ELBOWS.

Muscle ease balm

WARM CINNAMON AND COOL PEPPERMINT MAKE THIS AN IDEAL MASSAGE BALM TO HELP EASE TENSE AND TIRED MUSCLES. USE SPARINGLY ON LOCALIZED AREAS WHERE MUSCLES ARE TENSE AND NEED SOME EXTRA TLC!

MAKES 75 ML

10 g beeswax
60 ml grapeseed oil
15 ml coconut oil
8 drops rosemary essential oil
15 drops peppermint essential oil
10 drops eucalyptus essential oil
10 drops lavender essential oil
8 drops cinnamon essential oil

1. Melt the beeswax, grapeseed oil and coconut oil in a saucepan over low heat.
2. Once the oils and wax are completely melted, remove from the heat and stir in the essential oils.
3. Pour into a sterilized glass jar or plastic container to set.

How do I use the balm? This balm is very concentrated so use sparingly! Apply a small amount to areas needing pain relief and massage gently. This works very well as an application to ease muscular aches and pains in the neck, or to ease joint pain.

Revitalizing balm

PEPPERMINT, SPEARMINT AND LEMONGRASS OILS ARE REVITALIZING AND REFRESHING. THIS IS A WINNING COMBINATION FOR EASING HEAVY, TIRED LEGS DURING THE HOT SUMMER MONTHS, AND CAN ALSO BE USED AS A FOOT MASSAGE BALM.

MAKES 75 ML

10 g beeswax
60 ml grapeseed oil
15 ml coconut oil
8 drops peppermint essential oil
5 drops spearmint essential oil
5 drops lemon essential oil
3 drops lemongrass essential oil

1. Melt the beeswax, grapeseed oil and coconut oil in a saucepan over low heat.
2. Once the oils and wax are completely melted, remove from the heat and stir in the essential oils.
3. Pour into a sterilized glass jar or plastic container to set.

Rose garden balm

ROSE GERANIUM, ROSE AND YLANG YLANG OILS ARE RELAXING AND SOOTHING.

MAKES 75 ML

10 g beeswax
60 ml grapeseed oil
15 ml coconut oil
8 drops rose geranium essential oil
5 drops rose essential oil
4 drops ylang ylang essential oil

1. Melt the beeswax, grapeseed oil and coconut oil in a saucepan over low heat.
2. Once the oils and wax are completely melted, remove from the heat and stir in the essential oils.
3. Pour into a sterilized glass jar or plastic container to set.

Rose garden balm

Massage and bath oils

THESE OIL RECIPES CAN BE USED FOR AROMATHERAPY MASSAGE OR AROMATHERAPY BATHS. ADD 5 ML/1 TEASPOON TO A WARM BATH FOR A THERAPEUTIC AROMATHERAPY HOME SPA TREATMENT.

De-stress massage oil

ROSE GERANIUM IS REPUTED TO HAVE A BALANCING EFFECT ON THE BODY, HELPING COPE WITH STRESS AND THE DEMANDS OF A BUSY LIFESTYLE. FRANKINCENSE ESSENTIAL OIL IS OFTEN USED IN MEDITATION AND CAN HELP TO INDUCE RELAXATION BY CALMING THE NERVOUS SYSTEM. ORANGE ESSENTIAL OIL HELPS TO UPLIFT THE BODY AND SOUL.

MAKES 100 ML

1. Mix the oils together in a container and shake well.

100 ml sweet almond oil
15 drops rose geranium essential oil
6 drops frankincense essential oil
8 drops orange essential oil

Peace massage oil

THIS ESSENTIAL OIL BLEND IS A WINNING COMBINATION OF RELAXING ESSENTIAL OILS – CALMING LAVENDER AND NEROLI – KNOWN AS THE 'RESCUE REMEDY' OF THE ESSENTIAL OILS, AND VETIVER OIL, KNOWN AS THE 'OIL OF TRANQUILITY'.

MAKES 100 ML

1. Mix the oils together in a container and shake well.

100 ml sweet almond oil
12 drops lavender essential oil
8 drops neroli essential oil
5 drops vetiver essential oil

Sensual massage oil

RELAX AND UNWIND WITH THIS SENSUOUS BLEND OF OILS. YLANG YLANG AND PATCHOULI ARE REPUTED TO HAVE APHRODISIAC PROPERTIES, WHILE NEROLI ESSENTIAL OIL MAY HELP TO RELIEVE TENSION AND STRESS.

MAKES 100 ML

1. Mix the oils together in a container and shake well.

100 ml sweet almond oil
8 drops ylang ylang essential oil
8 drops patchouli essential oil
6 drops neroli essential oil

De-stress massage oil

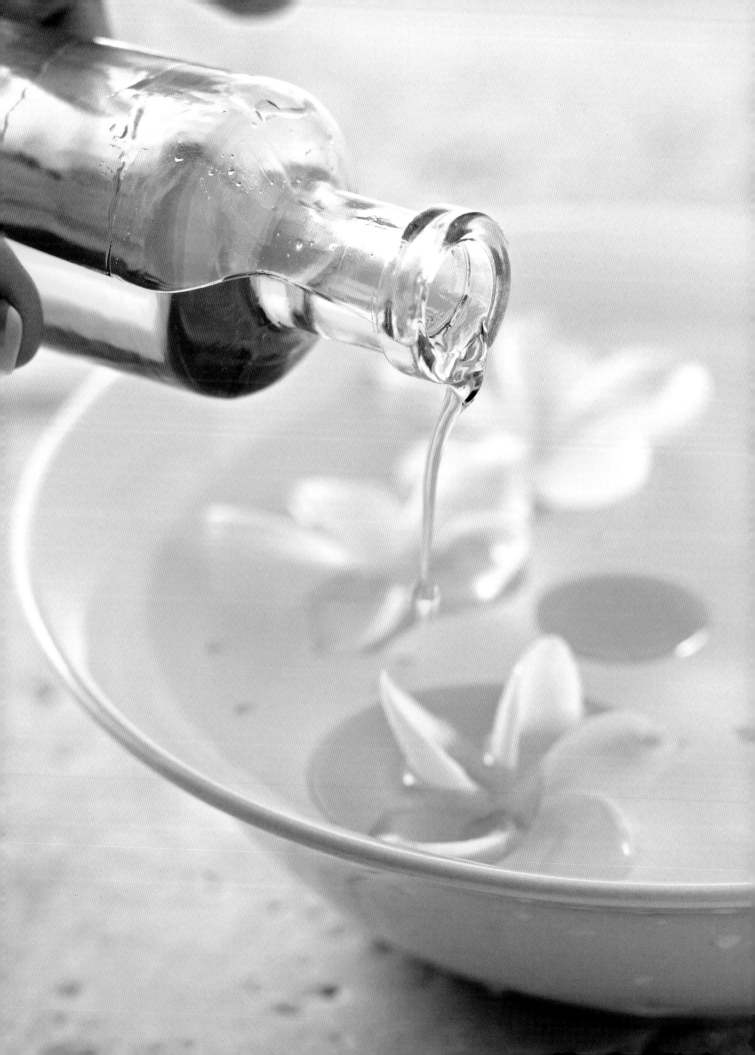

Products
for hands and feet

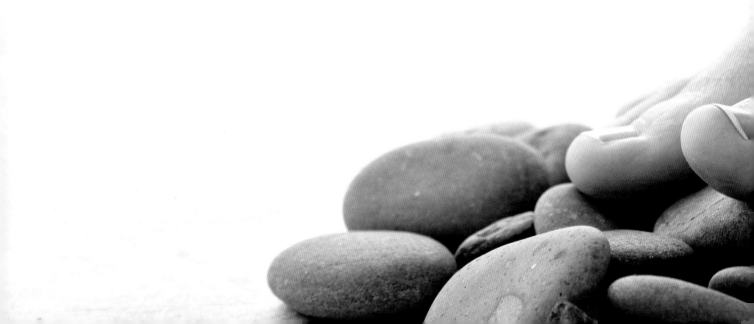

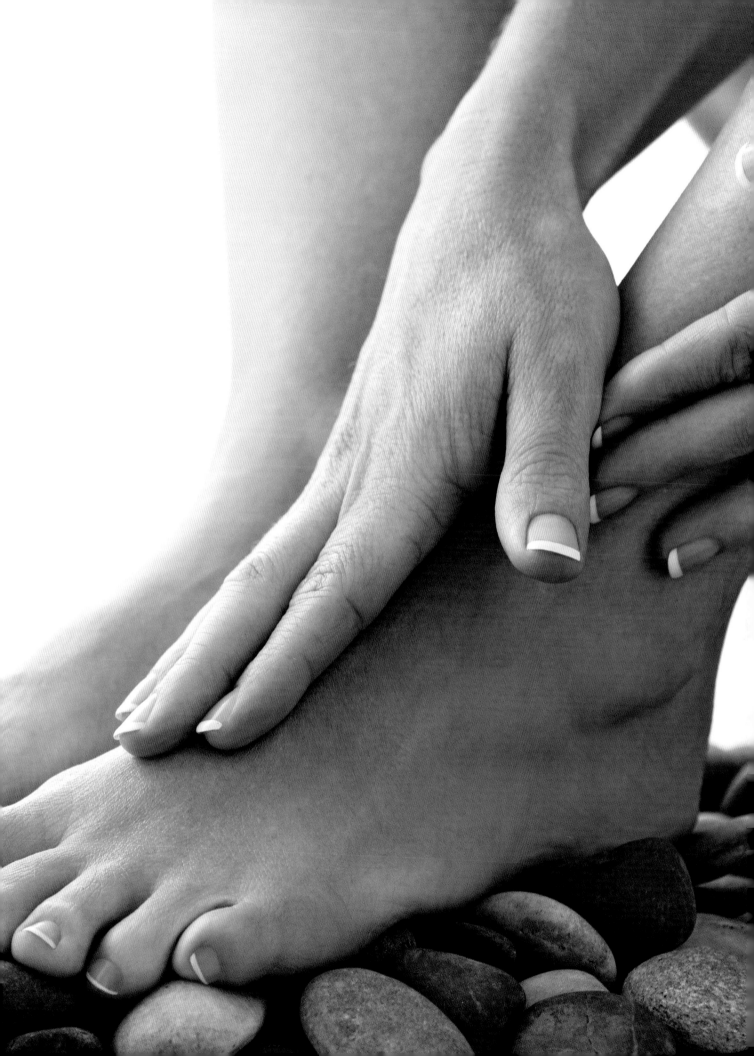

Moisturizing hand scrub

THE EXFOLIATING ALOE GEL AND CARRIER CREAM ARE READY-TO-USE, UNFRAGRANCED BASE PRODUCTS. SIMPLY MIX ALL OF THE INGREDIENTS TOGETHER AND CREATE YOUR OWN SPA MANICURE TREATMENT AT HOME! PALMAROSA AND LAVENDER ESSENTIAL OILS HAVE SKIN REGENERATING PROPERTIES, WHILE ROSE GERANIUM IS FRESH AND ROSY, AND IS WELL KNOWN FOR ITS USE IN MANY SKIN CARE PREPARATIONS.

MAKES 250 ML

100 ml exfoliating aloe gel
125 ml carrier cream
10 ml neem oil
10 ml jojoba oil
5 drops palmarosa essential oil
6 drops rose geranium essential oil
5 drops mandarin essential oil
4 drops grapefruit essential oil

1. Mix the exfoliating aloe gel and carrier cream together.
2. Add the neem and jojoba oils and mix until the oils have been incorporated into the cream mixture.
3. Add the essential oils and mix well.
4. Spoon into sterilized glass or plastic containers.

How do I use the hand scrub? Soak your hands in a bowl of warm water for about 1 minute. Remove your hands from the bowl of water and pat dry. Apply 15 ml moisturizing hand scrub and massage gently into the hands and cuticles. Return your hands to the bowl of warm water and rinse off. Dry your hands well, and then follow with an application of Cuticle Oil (see page 39) to the cuticles.

Luxurious hand cream

A RICH FORMULA FOR TREATING DRY SKIN AND STRENGTHENING THE NAILS, AND FOR KEEPING THE HANDS SOFT AND SILKY.

MAKES 300 ML

100 ml shea butter
200 ml carrier cream
20 ml jojoba oil
8 drops neroli essential oil
6 drops lavender essential oil
4 drops patchouli essential oil

1. Melt the shea butter in a saucepan over very gentle heat.
2. Place the shea butter in the fridge until it solidifies again and is the consistency of soft butter. (The reason for doing this is that sometimes when incorporating shea butter into creams and lotions, the product becomes grainy in texture. This is due to the changes in temperature, and by re-melting the shea butter, it remains more stable.)
3. In a separate bowl, mix the carrier cream and jojoba oil until the oil is incorporated.
4. Add the essential oils and mix well.
5. Once the shea butter has returned to a solid state, slowly add the carrier cream mixture to the shea butter, and mix with a whisk until combined.
6. Spoon into sterilized glass or plastic containers.

How do I use the hand cream? Apply to cleansed hands and gently massage into the nails for a moisturizing hand treatment.

Luxurious hand cream

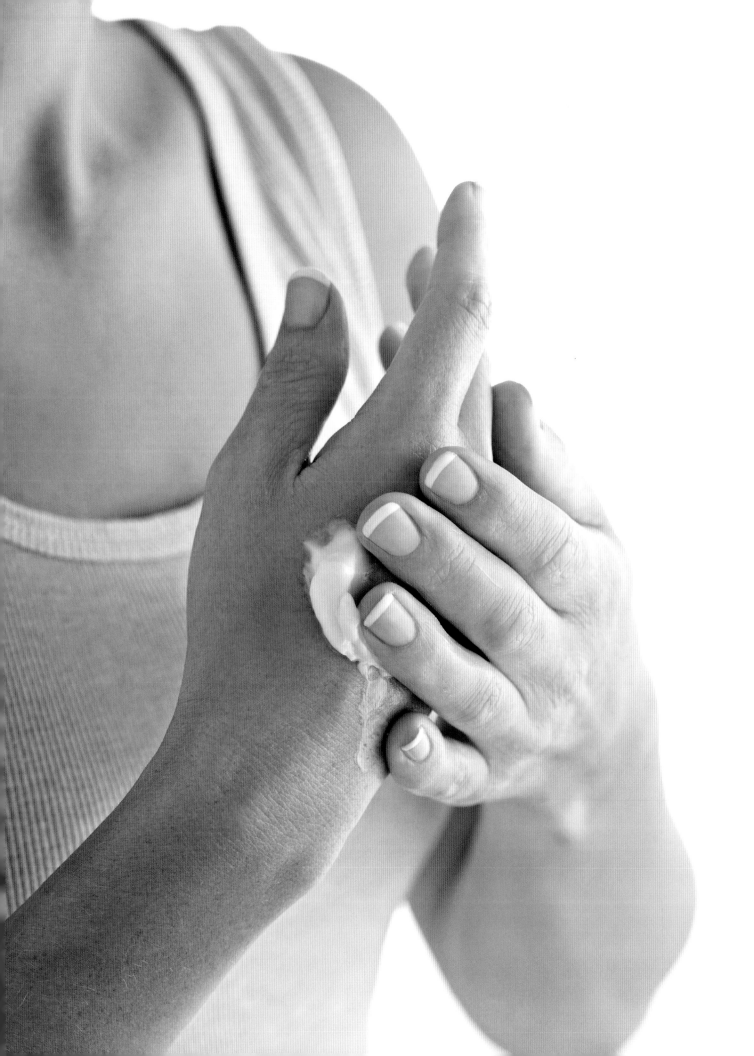

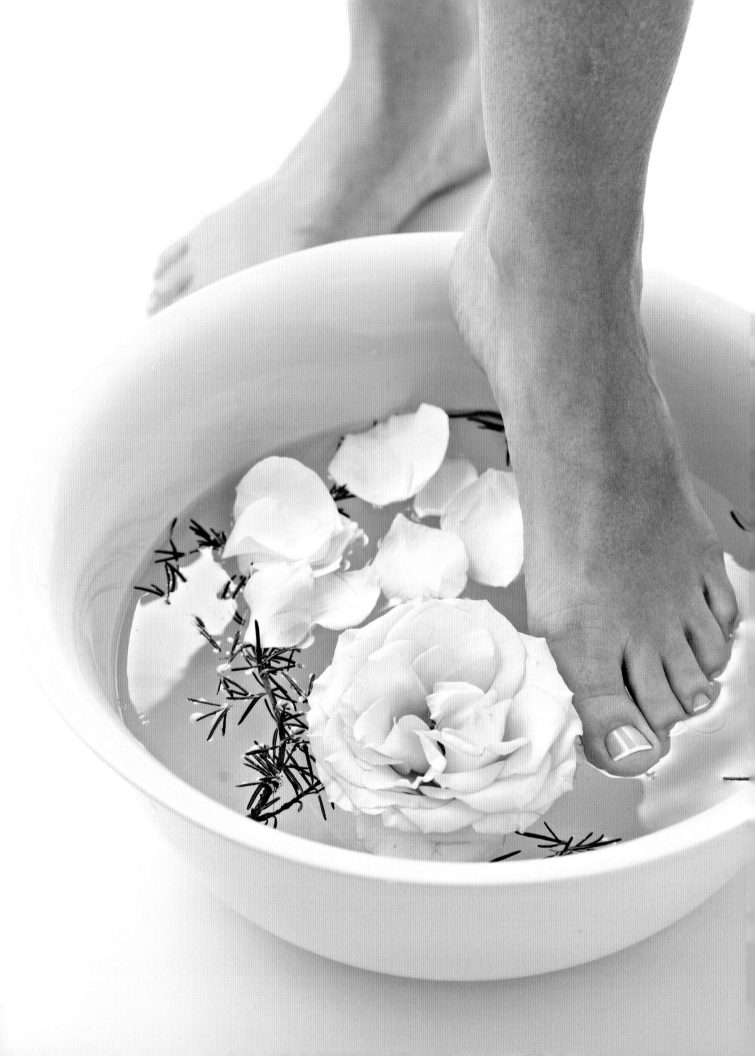

Cuticle oil

SWEET ALMOND AND NEEM OILS SOFTEN AND MOISTURIZE THE SKIN AROUND THE NAILS, WHILE PROVIDING NUTRIENTS TO THE CUTICLE AREA. ESSENTIAL OILS OF LAVENDER, TEA TREE AND ROSE GERANIUM HAVE ANTI-FUNGAL PROPERTIES, WHICH CAN HELP TO PREVENT INFECTIOUS NAIL CONDITIONS.

MAKES 50 ML

30 ml sweet almond oil
20 ml neem oil
2 drops lavender essential oil
1 drop tea tree essential oil
1 drop rose geranium essential oil

1. Combine the sweet almond oil and neem oil in a sterilized glass or plastic bottle.
2. Add the essential oils and shake well.

How do I use the cuticle oil? Apply to cleansed hands and feet. Massage gently into the cuticles of the nails.

Relaxing rosemary, lavender and tea tree foot soak

BICARBONATE OF SODA SOFTENS THE WATER AND ROSEMARY, LAVENDER AND TEA TREE ESSENTIAL OILS PACK A POWERFUL PUNCH AGAINST FUNGAL INFECTIONS. THIS FOOT SOAK IS PERFECT FOR HARD, DRY SKIN AND CRACKED HEELS OR SIMPLY JUST TO SOOTHE TIRED FEET AFTER A HARD DAY'S WORK.

MAKES 250 ML

250 ml bicarbonate of soda
5 drops rosemary essential oil
5 drops lavender essential oil
5 drops tea tree essential oil
50 ml dried lavender flowers

1. Place the bicarbonate of soda and essential oils together in a mixing bowl and mix well.
2. Crush the dried lavender flowers and sprinkle over the bicarbonate of soda mixture. Mix well to incorporate the essential oils.

How do I use the foot soak? Add 50 ml foot soak mixture to warm water in a foot bath and soak your feet for a few minutes. Towel dry and follow with the Exfoliating Minty Foot Scrub (see page 40).

Relaxing rosemary, lavender and tea tree foot soak

Exfoliating minty foot scrub

I LOVE TO USE THIS FOOT SCRUB AFTER MY FEET HAVE BEEN SOAKING IN WATER CONTAINING SOME OF THE ROSEMARY, LAVENDER AND TEA TREE FOOT SOAK (SEE PAGE 39). TOWEL DRY YOUR FEET AND MASSAGE AWAY ALL THE ROUGH SKIN. THIS SCRUB IS GENTLER THAN SALT SCRUBS AND CAN ALSO BE USED ON YOUR LEGS.

MAKES 250 ML

150 ml exfoliating aloe gel
100 ml carrier cream
10 ml olive oil
10 drops peppermint essential oil
8 drops spearmint essential oil
5 drops tea tree essential oil

1. Mix the exfoliating aloe gel and carrier cream together.
2. Add the olive oil and mix until the oil is incorporated.
3. Add the essential oils and mix well.
4. Spoon into a sterilized glass or plastic jar.

How do I use the foot scrub? Soak your feet in a foot bath of warm water for about 5 minutes. Towel dry. Apply 15 ml exfoliating scrub per foot, and massage gently into your feet. Return your feet to the foot bath to rinse. Towel dry your feet (dry between your toes to prevent fungal infections) and apply Refreshing Lemongrass and Spearmint Foot Cream (see page 43).

Cinnamon and coffee foot mask

THIS MASK SMELLS ABSOLUTELY DELICIOUS. COFFEE, CINNAMON AND CLAY FORM THE BASE OF THIS FOOT TREATMENT, AND THESE INGREDIENTS HELP TO RINSE AWAY DEAD SKIN CELLS AND EXFOLIATE AT THE SAME TIME. IT IS A BIT OF A MESSY PROCEDURE, BUT WELL WORTH IT.

MAKES 200 ML

120 ml kaolin clay powder
15 ml ground cinnamon
15 ml ground coffee beans
50 ml warm water
6 drops sandalwood essential oil
3 drops ginger essential oil

1. Place the kaolin clay powder, cinnamon and ground coffee in a bowl and mix together.
2. Add the warm water and essential oils and mix well until you have a smooth clay paste. If the mixture is too dry, simply add a little more warm water until you have the desired consistency. If the mixture is too runny, add a little more kaolin clay powder.

How do I use the foot mask? Soak your feet in a foot bath of warm water for about 5 minutes. Towel dry. Apply to cleansed feet and allow to dry for about 5 minutes. To remove the mask, soak 2 muslin cloths (or large facecloths) in warm water and wrap the warm cloths around your feet. Remove the mask by gently wiping off most of the clay. You may need to repeat this process several times to ensure that all residue of the mask is removed properly.
Alternatively: Prepare a foot bath with warm water and soak your feet to remove the foot mask.

Cinnamon and coffee foot mask

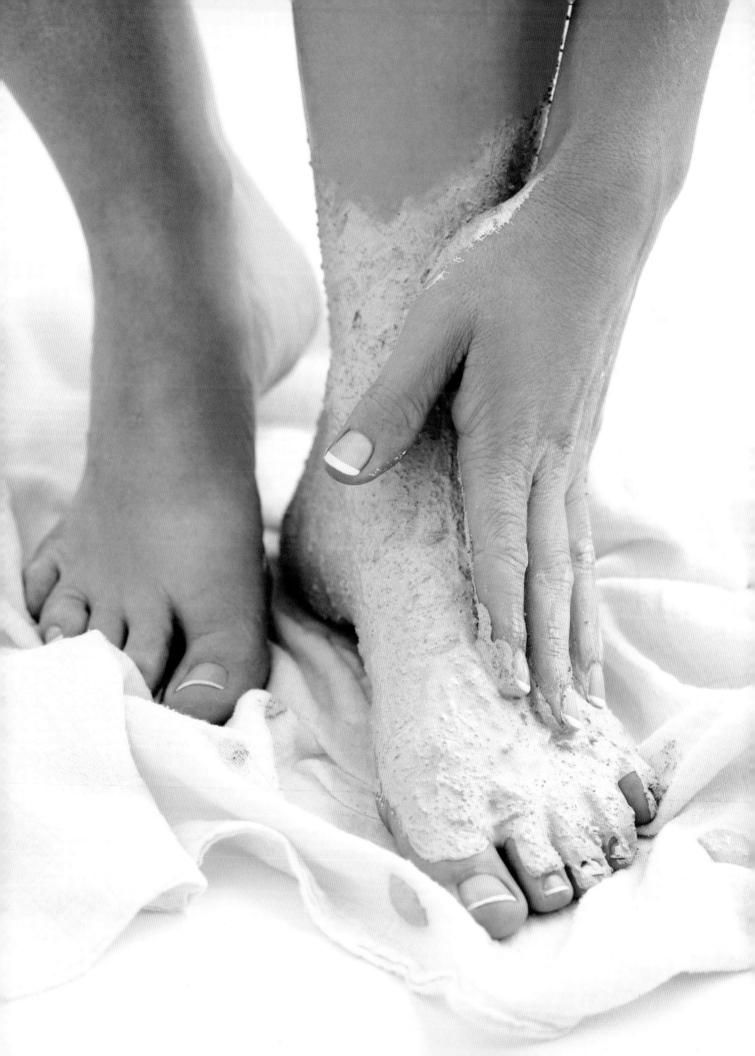

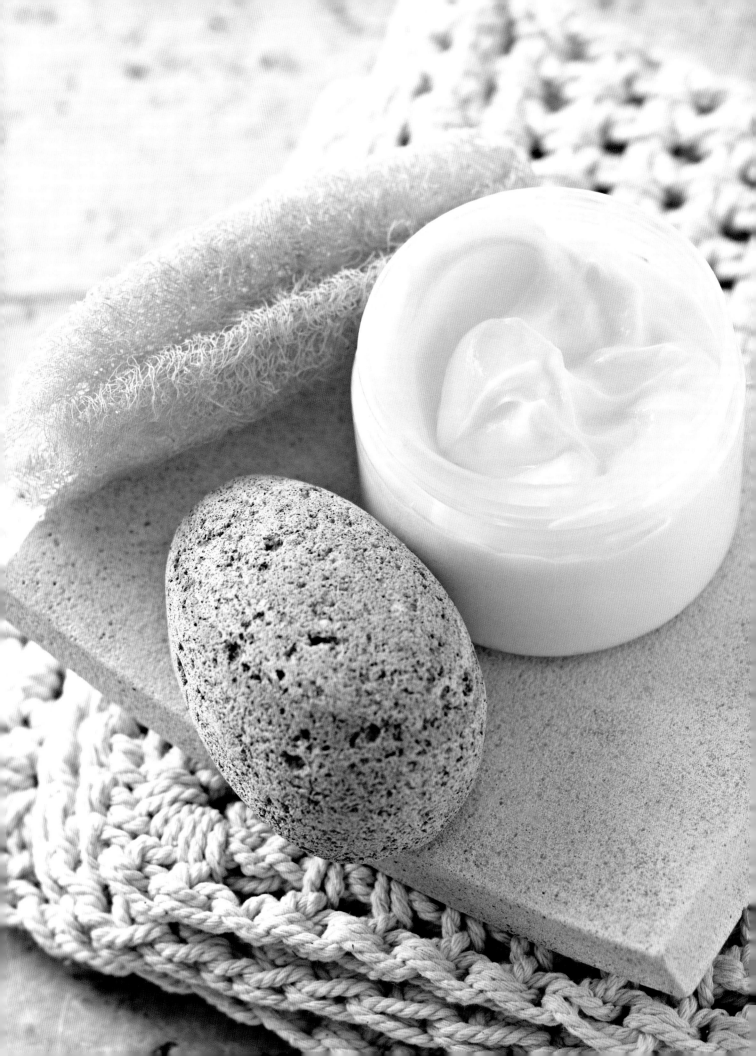

Refreshing lemongrass and spearmint foot cream

CREAMY, MOISTURIZING AND FRESH! THIS FOOT CREAM CAN ALSO BE USED TO GENTLY MASSAGE THE LEGS (I FIND IT VERY USEFUL IN COMBATING DRY SKIN ON THE LOWER LEGS). SPEARMINT ESSENTIAL OIL IS GENTLE, BUT ALSO HAS A WONDERFULLY COOLING SENSATION ON THE LEGS. THE LEMONGRASS AND LEMON ESSENTIAL OILS PROVIDE A ZINGY, FRESH AROMA.

MAKES 250 ML

250 ml thickened carrier cream
20 ml olive oil
6 drops lemongrass essential oil
4 drops lemon essential oil
8 drops spearmint essential oil

1. Place the carrier cream and olive oil in a mixing bowl and whisk together until combined.
2. Add the essential oils and mix well.
3. Spoon the mixture into sterilized glass or plastic jars.

How do I use the foot cream? Apply liberally to cleansed feet as a nourishing foot cream, to prevent dry and cracked heels.

 Tip: Apply a generous amount of foot cream to cleansed feet and wear thick, comfortable socks. This will help the cream to penetrate the skin, resulting in smooth, silky feet.

Smoothing foot treatment mask for dry and cracked heels

CONTAINS NOURISHING SHEA BUTTER, AS WELL AS THE ESSENTIAL OILS OF PALMAROSA AND ORANGE, WHICH PROVIDE A PLEASANT FRUITY SCENT. FRANKINCENSE (WHICH IS EXTRACTED FROM THE GUM OR RESIN OF A SMALL AFRICAN SHRUB) IS INDICATED FOR ITS USE ON VERY DRY SKIN AND CAN HELP TO HEAL AND REPAIR CHAPPED SKIN.

MAKES 250 ML

100 ml shea butter
100 ml thickened carrier cream
50 ml sweet almond oil or grapeseed oil
6 drops palmarosa essential oil
6 drops frankincense essential oil
8 drops orange or mandarin
  essential oil

1. Melt the shea butter in a saucepan over very gentle heat.
2. Place the shea butter in the fridge until it solidifies again (and is the consistency of soft butter).
3. In a separate bowl, mix together the carrier cream and sweet almond or grapeseed oil until combined.
4. Add the essential oils and mix well.
5. Once the shea butter has returned to a solid state, slowly add the carrier cream to the shea butter and mix with a whisk until combined.
6. Spoon into sterilized glass or plastic containers.

How do I use the foot mask? Soak feet using the Relaxing Rosemary, Lavender and Tea Tree Foot Soak (see page 39). Dry feet thoroughly and apply about 5 ml treatment mask to each foot, massaging it into the feet. Wrap each foot in a hand towel and allow the mask to work into the skin. Leave for approximately 10 minutes. Either massage the remaining mask into the feet or wipe off any residue with the towel if it feels too oily.

Refreshing lemongrass and spearmint foot cream

Hair products

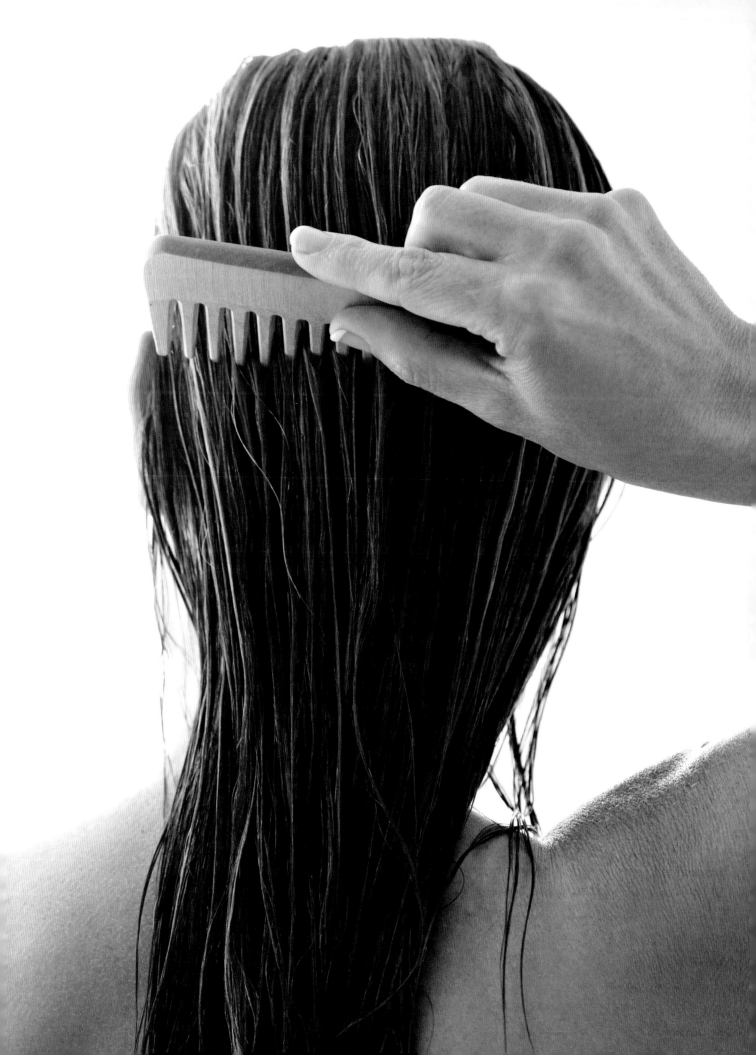

Rosemary, peppermint and orange shampoo

THIS INVIGORATING HAIR SHAMPOO IS LOW IN SULPHATES AND IS GENTLE ON THE SCALP. JOJOBA OIL HELPS TO MOISTURIZE AND CONDITION THE HAIR, WHILE ROSEMARY AND PEPPERMINT ARE STIMULATING AND REFRESHING.

MAKES 225 ML

200 ml surfactant base
10 ml filtered water
10 ml jojoba oil
8 drops rosemary essential oil
4 drops peppermint essential oil
8 drops orange essential oil

1. Mix all the ingredients together in a jug and stir well until combined. Decant into a plastic container.
2. Wet hair and use a small amount of shampoo. Lather into the hair and then rinse well. Follow with a herbal conditioning rinse (see page 49).

Coconut, ylang ylang and patchouli hair mask

RESTORE YOUR LUSCIOUS LOCKS WITH THIS AGE-OLD RECIPE. THE INDONESIANS ALSO MAKE HOME-MADE HAIR CONDITIONERS AND LEAVE-IN HAIR TREATMENTS WITH COCONUT OIL. IN THE VICTORIAN AND EDWARDIAN ERAS IT BECAME SO POPULAR TO CONDITION THE HAIR WITH LEAVE-IN HAIR CONDITIONERS, CALLED MACASSAR OIL, THAT HOUSEWIVES STARTED DRAPING PROTECTIVE CLOTHS OVER THE FURNITURE TO PREVENT THE FABRIC FROM BEING RUINED BY THE OILS. THESE OLD-FASHIONED DOILIES BECAME KNOWN AS ANTIMACASSARS. IF YOU INTEND TO USE THIS MASK AS AN OVERNIGHT TREATMENT, REMEMBER TO USE AN OLD PILLOWCASE.

MAKES 150 ML

50 ml coconut oil
100 ml sweet almond oil
3 drops ylang ylang essential oil
3 drops patchouli essential oil

1. Melt the coconut oil and almond oil together in a saucepan over low heat. Once the oils have melted, remove from the heat.
2. Stir in the essential oils.
3. Pour into a plastic tub or glass container.

How do I use the hair mask? Wet hair and apply a handful of hair mask. Massage the mask into the scalp and hair. Cover the hair with a shower cap (or a little plastic wrap, wrapped loosely around the hair) and wrap your head in a small towel for about 30 minutes, or even overnight! Shampoo twice and follow with a herbal conditioning rinse (see page 49).

Tip: Heat the towel in some warm water and wring it out well. Use the heated towel to wrap around your head. The heat will help the nourishing oils penetrate the hair and scalp.

Rosemary, peppermint and orange shampoo and
Coconut, ylang ylang and patchouli hair mask

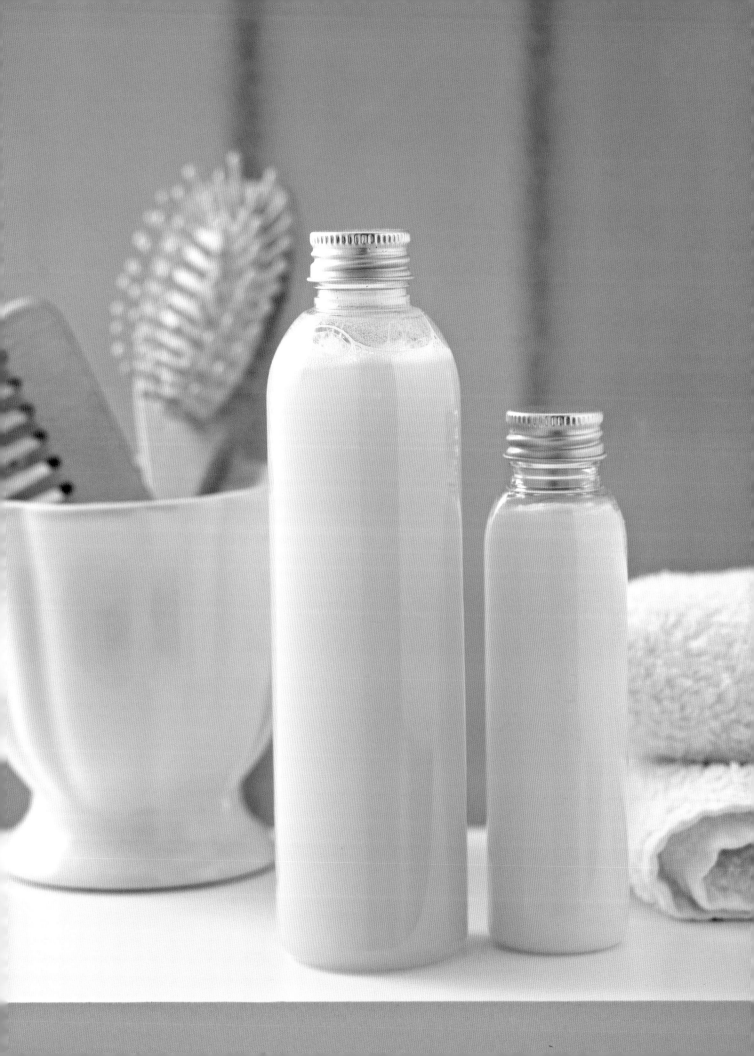

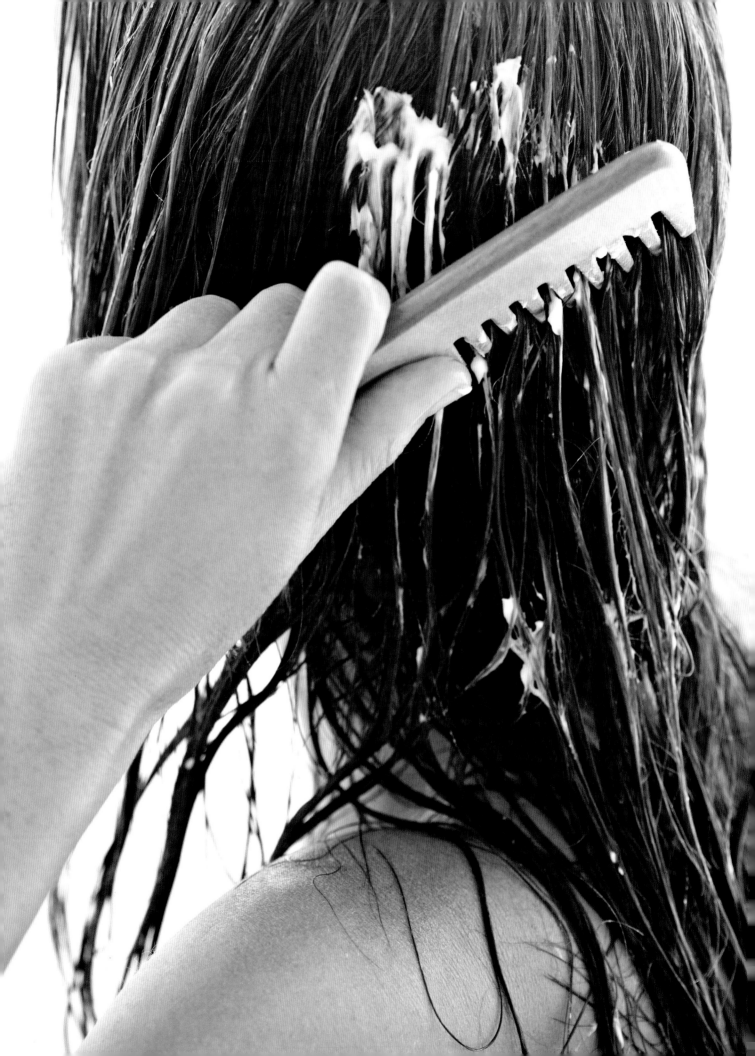

Shimmering hair mask

ARGAN OIL ORIGINATES FROM MOROCCO. THIS OIL, EXTRACTED FROM THE NUTS OF A DESERT TREE, IS A GOOD CONDITIONER FOR THE SKIN AND HAIR, CREATING PROTECTION AND SHINE WITHOUT LEAVING A HEAVY RESIDUE. JOJOBA OIL IS USEFUL IN BALANCING DRY AND OILY SKIN, AND PROVIDES EXTRA MOISTURE FOR THE SCALP AND HAIR FOLLICLES. THE OIL CAN ALSO BE USED AS A CONDITIONING TREATMENT FOR ALL DAY USE. ADD A FEW DROPS TO CLEAN, DRY HAIR AND MASSAGE GENTLY INTO THE SCALP AND THE REST OF THE HAIR. COMB THROUGH WITH A WIDE-TOOTHED COMB.

MAKES 150 ML

40 ml coconut oil
10 ml shea butter
50 ml argan oil
50 ml jojoba oil
1 drop rose geranium essential oil
1 drop fennel essential oil

1. Melt the coconut oil and shea butter in a saucepan over gentle heat. Pour all the ingredients into a glass bottle or plastic container and shake well.

How do I use the hair mask? Wet hair and apply a handful of hair mask. Massage the mask into the scalp and hair. Cover the hair with a shower cap (or a little plastic wrap, wrapped loosely around the hair) and wrap your head in a small towel for about 30 minutes, or even overnight! Shampoo twice and follow with a herbal conditioning rinse (see below).

Chamomile and orange blossom conditioning rinse (for blonde hair)

NATURAL HAIR RINSES CONTAINING VINEGAR CAN HELP REMOVE EXCESS OIL RESIDUE ON THE SCALP, LEAVING THE HAIR SOFT AND SHINY. CHAMOMILE TEA HAS BEEN USED THROUGHOUT THE AGES AS A TONIC AND TREATMENT FOR BLONDE OR LIGHT HAIR, AND CAN ALSO HELP TO SUPPLY NUTRIENTS AND VITALITY.

MAKES 250 ML (ENOUGH FOR 2 APPLICATIONS)

250 ml boiling water
1 chamomile tea bag
5 ml apple cider vinegar
1 drop neroli essential oil (optional)

1. Pour the boiling water over the chamomile tea bag and steep for 10 minutes.
2. Add the vinegar and essential oil and mix well.
3. Allow to cool slightly. The mixture can be warm when you use it, but make sure that it is not too hot when you rinse your hair!

How do I use the conditioning rinse? Shampoo hair with herbal shampoo and rinse well. Rinse your hair with 125 ml conditioning herbal rinse, and do not rinse out of the hair. Towel dry and style hair as usual.

Rosemary and geranium conditioning rinse (for dark hair)

ROSEMARY IS AN EXCELLENT HAIR TONIC AND IS OFTEN USED IN HAIR TREATMENTS TO STIMULATE THE SCALP AND PROMOTE HAIR GROWTH.

MAKES 250 ML (ENOUGH FOR 2 APPLICATIONS)

250 ml boiling water
30 ml dried rosemary or 2 large fresh rosemary sprigs
5 ml apple cider vinegar
1 drop geranium essential oil (optional)

1. Pour the boiling water over the rosemary and steep for 10 minutes.
2. Add the apple cider vinegar and essential oil and mix well.
3. Allow to cool slightly. The mixture can be warm, but make sure that it is not too hot when you rinse your hair!

How do I use the conditioning rinse? Shampoo hair with herbal shampoo and rinse well. Rinse your hair with 125 ml conditioning herbal rinse, and do not rinse out of the hair. Towel dry and style hair as usual.

Shimmering hair mask

Bath products

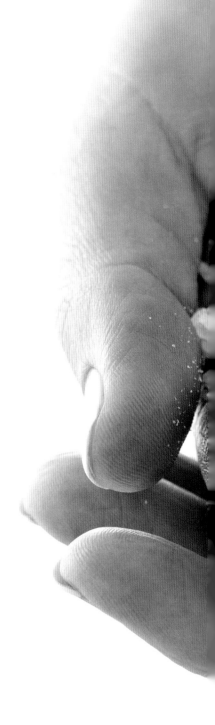

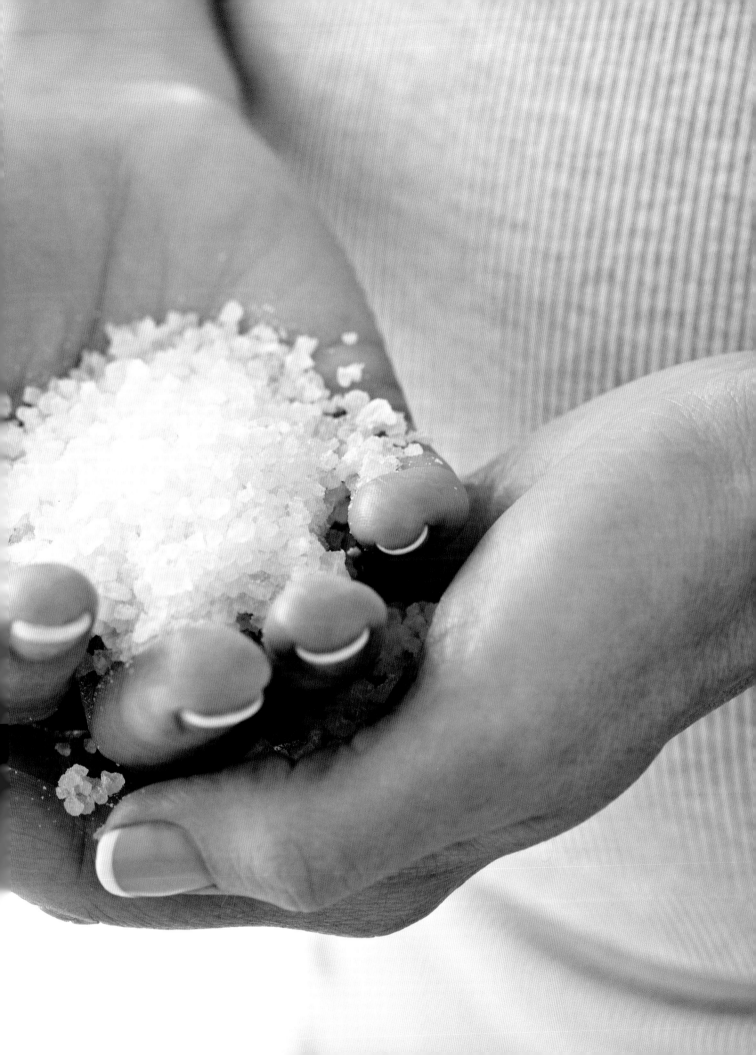

Rose petal bath fizz balls

THESE BATH FIZZ BALLS ARE GREAT FUN TO MAKE. ROSE PETALS AND ROSE GERANIUM ESSENTIAL OIL GIVE THE FIZZ BALLS A SUBTLE ROSE AROMA AND THEY LOOK STUNNING WHEN USING DARK RED ROSE PETALS. (WHITE OR LIGHT PINK PETALS TEND TO TURN A BIT BROWN WHEN ADDED TO THE FIZZ BALL MIXTURE.)

MAKES 8–10

500 g bicarbonate of soda
100 g citric acid
50 ml dried rose petals (torn into small pieces)
30 drops rose geranium essential oil
30–60 ml filtered water

1. Place the bicarbonate of soda and citric acid together in a plastic bowl.
2. Mix and crush the powder with a metal spoon until lump free.
3. Add the dried rose petals and essential oil and mix.
4. Add 30 ml of the water and mix, stirring and crushing the mixture with the spoon until you have the consistency of wet sand. Add more water if needed.
5. Scoop a generous amount of mixture into each half of the empty table tennis balls and push them together. Squeeze to combine the two halves.
6. Carefully remove each half of the table tennis balls and place the bath fizz balls on a dishcloth to dry out. Once the fizz balls have hardened completely and are safe to handle, place them in empty egg trays to dry.
7. The fizz balls will be dry within an hour – package and decorate as you like!

How do I use the bath fizz balls? Add 1 bath fizz ball to your bath water or try using a bath fizz ball in your foot spa water for an extra treat.

Tip: Keep your red roses after they are no longer suitable for display in a vase. Remove the petals from the stems and place onto newspaper. Set aside for a few days until completely dry, and then store them in a glass jar or airtight plastic container.

Lavender flower bath fizzies

THESE BATH FIZZ BALLS ARE REALLY EASY TO MAKE AND THE PURPLE LAVENDER FLOWERS LOOK SO PRETTY!

MAKES ABOUT 24, DEPENDING ON SIZE

500 g bicarbonate of soda
100 g citric acid
50 ml dried lavender flowers
30 drops lavender essential oil
30–60 ml filtered water

1. Place the bicarbonate of soda and citric acid together in a plastic bowl.
2. Mix and crush the powder with a metal spoon until lump free.
3. Add the dried lavender flowers and essential oil and mix again.
4. Add 30 ml of the water and mix very well, stirring and crushing the mixture with the metal spoon until you have the consistency of wet sand. Add more water if necessary.
5. Press into a soap mould or ice-cube trays and allow to dry for 30 minutes.
6. Turn the mould upside down and give it a tap to release the bath fizzies.

Try these variations for bath fizz balls or bath fizzies:

Lemon rose: rose and calendula petals with 20 drops rose geranium essential oil and 10 drops lemon essential oil
Spicy orange: 2.5 ml ground cinnamon with 25 drops orange essential oil and 4 drops cinnamon essential oil
Chamomile orange: 5 ml dried chamomile flowers with 25 drops orange essential oil and 5 drops mandarin essential oil
Herbal: 5 ml dried rosemary with 20 drops rosemary essential oil and 10 drops peppermint essential oil

Tip: If you don't have dried lavender flowers you can use any dried herbs (rosemary, oregano, basil, etc.) instead. To dry your own lavender, pick plenty of fresh lavender when the flowers are in abundance. Pick the top purple parts of the lavender stalks and flowers and rub off the stem. Place onto a sheet of newspaper to dry for a few days and store in a glass jar or airtight plastic container.

*Rose petal bath fizz balls and
Lavender flower bath fizzies*

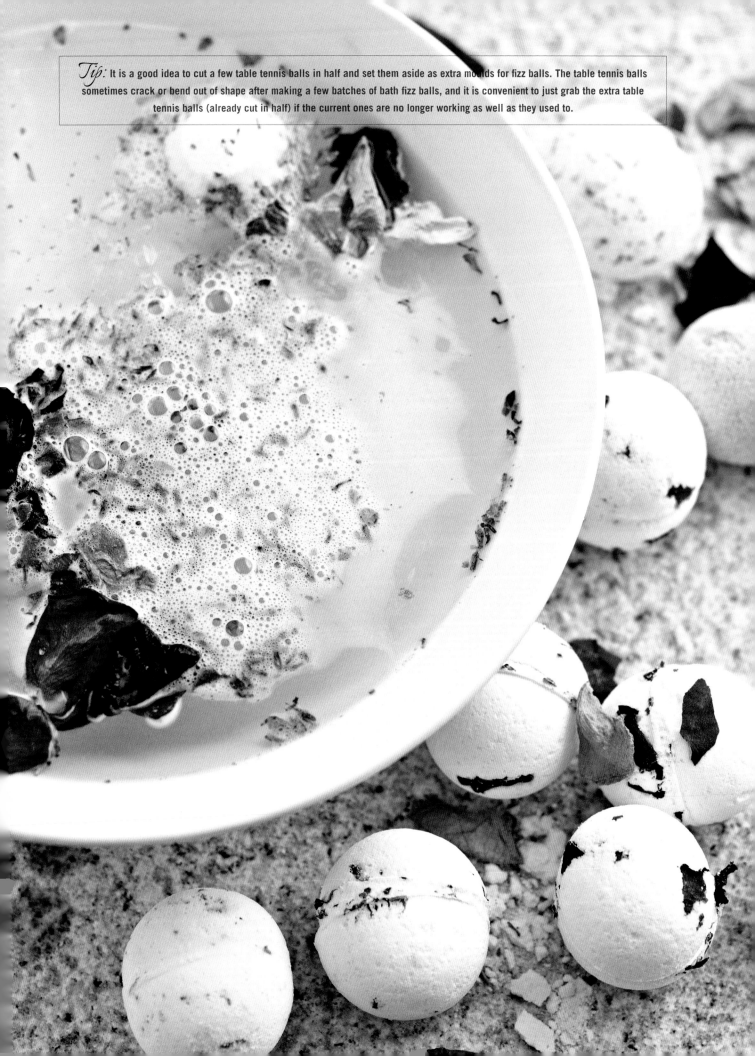

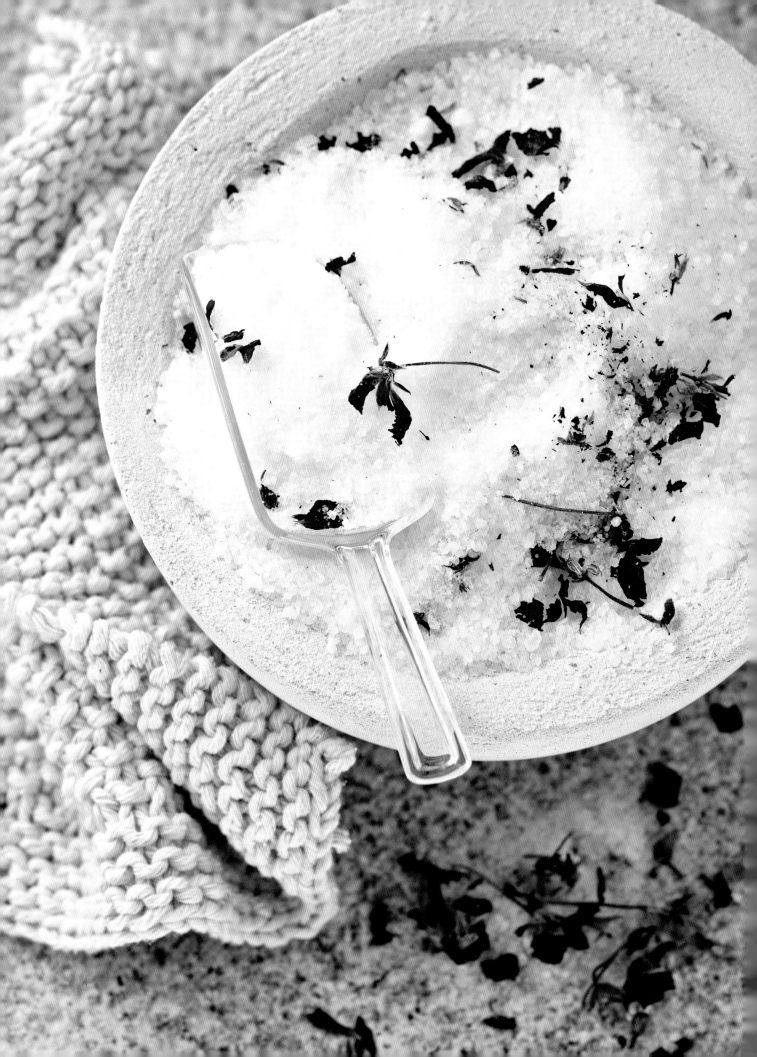

Cocoa butter bath melts with ylang ylang and patchouli

COCOA BUTTER IS THE OIL THAT HAS BEEN COLD-PRESSED FROM THE COCOA BEAN. IT IS AN IDEAL MOISTURIZER AND WHEN COMBINED WITH COCONUT OIL IT MAKES A VERY INTENSE TREATMENT FOR DRY SKIN. THIS IS A SPECIAL BATH TREAT WITH ESSENTIAL OILS OF YLANG YLANG, PATCHOULI AND LAVENDER TO CALM AND RELAX THE BODY, MIND AND SOUL.

MAKES ABOUT 8

50 g cocoa butter, finely grated
10 ml coconut oil
5 ml sunflower oil or grapeseed oil
6 drops ylang ylang essential oil
4 drops patchouli essential oil
6 drops lavender essential oil

1. Place the grated cocoa butter in a heatproof mixing bowl and suspend over a saucepan of simmering water. Do not let the water touch the bowl or get any water into the cocoa butter. Heat until the cocoa butter has melted.
2. Add the coconut oil, sunflower oil and then stir in the essential oils.
3. Pour into small chocolate moulds (I use tiny angel moulds) or you can also use silicone ice-cube trays.
4. Allow to set at room temperature for approximately 24 hours.
5. Allow to set completely before turning out.

How do I use the bath melts? Add 1 bath melt to a warm bath and it will dissolve into the bath water.

Bath sea salts

SUCH AN EASY RECIPE FOR A SPA TREAT, AND PERFECT FOR EVEN THE MOST UNDOMESTICATED GODDESS!

MAKES 250 ML

250 ml sea salt
handful of dried herbs or flowers
essential oils (see variations below)

1. Place all the ingredients together in a bowl and mix well.

How do I use the bath sea salts? Add a generous handful of bath salts to a warm bath, climb in and relax!

Tip: Try using the bath salts in a foot bath for an aromatherapy foot soak treatment. You will still have the wonderful aroma of the essential oils and the salt is cleansing and soothing for tired feet.

Variations – add the following essential oils:
Relax and de-stress: 10 drops rosewood, 6 drops geranium, 4 drops ginger
Peace: 10 drops lavender, 6 drops neroli, 5 drops vetiver
Rooibos: 8 drops grapefruit, 5 drops orange, 5 drops lemongrass, 6 drops mandarin, 2.5 ml rooibos extract

Bath sea salts

Magnesium bath crystals to relieve aching muscles

EPSOM SALTS (MAGNESIUM SULPHATE) BATHS HELP TO EASE MUSCLE TENSION BY DRAWING OUT ACIDIC WASTE FROM THE MUSCLES AND JOINTS THROUGH THE PORES OF THE SKIN. THIS MUSCLE SOAK TREATMENT IS REALLY HELPFUL TO RELEASE TENSION FROM TIRED AND OVERWORKED MUSCLES, ESPECIALLY SPORT-RELATED MUSCLE STIFFNESS. YOU CAN FIND EPSOM SALTS IN THE BAKING AISLE OF YOUR LOCAL SUPERMARKET.

MAKES 500 G

500 g Epsom salts
4 drops lavender essential oil
3 drops lemon essential oil
2 drops rosemary essential oil

1. Mix the Epsom salts and essential oils together and store in a plastic or glass container.

How do I use the bath crystals? Dissolve 250 ml of the bath crystals in warm water and add to a hot bath. Soak for at least 10 minutes in a warm bath as stiff muscles and joints respond well to heat. Afterwards, wear warm, comfortable clothes – or a gown – and allow a recovery period of at least 20 minutes. Drink at least 2 glasses of water during and/or after your spa bath treatment. If you suffer from arthritis and/or stiff joints, it is best to keep moving after your bath. Gentle stretches and exercises to stimulate the joints can be beneficial. Remember to relax afterwards.

Flu-buster and immune boosting magnesium bath crystals

EPSOM SALTS CAN ALSO BE USED TO RELAX SORE MUSCLES THAT OFTEN ACCOMPANY THE ONSET OF FLU. THE IMMUNE-STIMULATING ESSENTIAL OILS IN THESE BATH CRYSTALS WILL HELP TO EASE THE SYMPTOMS OF COLDS AND FLU. REMEMBER, REST AND RECOVERY IS VERY IMPORTANT WHEN YOU ARE TRYING TO FIGHT COLDS AND FLU.

MAKES 500 G

500 g Epsom salts
3 drops eucalyptus essential oil
2 drops pine essential oil
3 drops tea tree essential oil

1. Mix the Epsom salts and essential oils together and store in a plastic or glass container.

How do I use the bath crystals? Dissolve 250 ml of the bath crystals in warm water and add to a hot bath. Soak for at least 10 minutes in a warm bath as stiff muscles and joints respond well to heat. Afterwards, wear warm, comfortable clothes – or a gown – and allow a recovery period of at least 20 minutes. Enjoy a spa bath treatment daily for 3 days, and then every alternate day until the end of the week.

Tip: Remember to consult your local health care practitioner to assist you with herbal supplements and vitamins that can help you to recover faster. Vitamin C is recommended for periods of infection, and herbal extracts or tinctures of echinacea and goldenseal can also be beneficial in helping to boost the immune system.

Magnesium bath crystals to relieve aching muscles

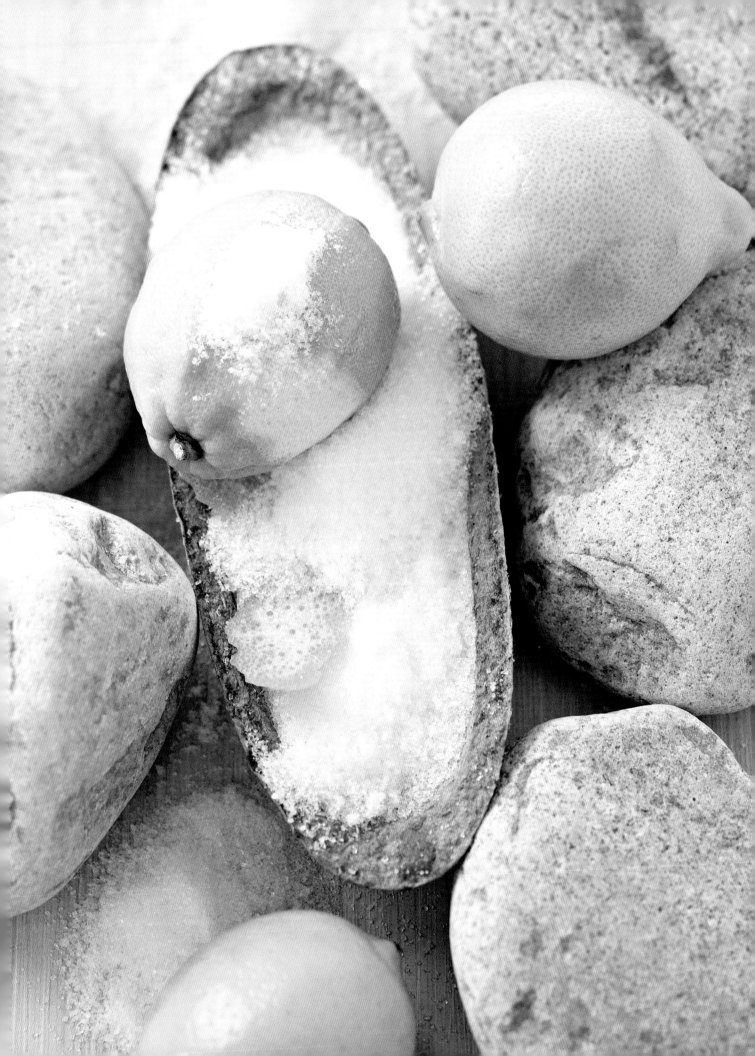

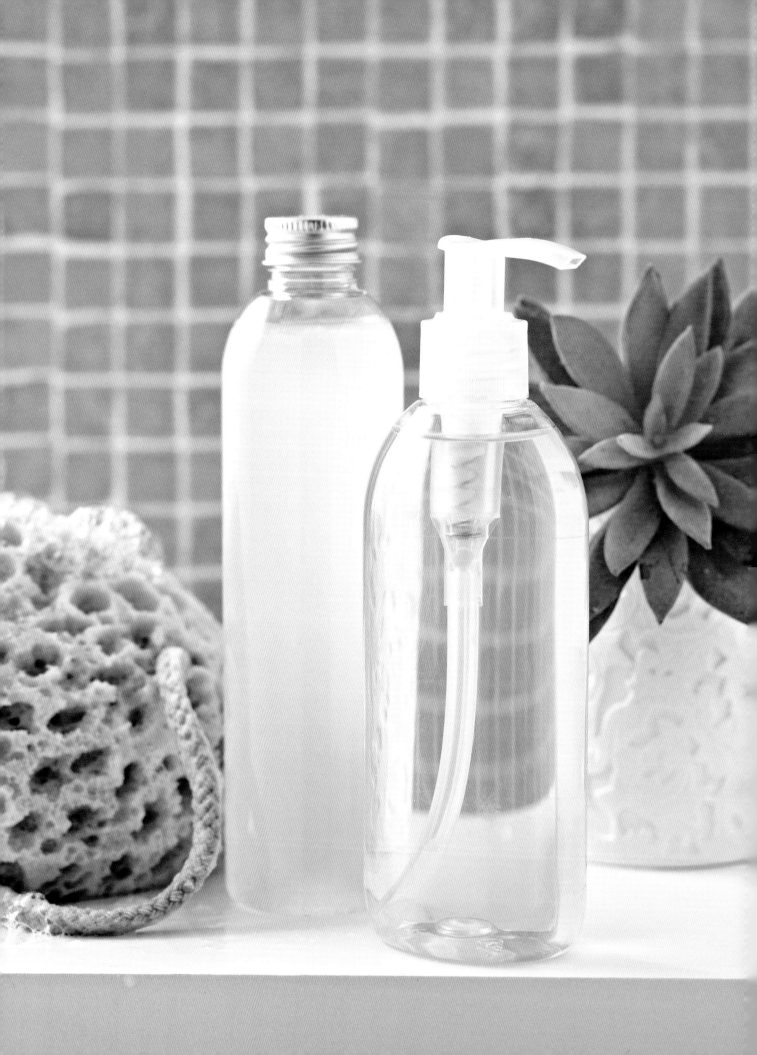

Foam bath or shower gels

THIS RECIPE USES AN UNFRAGRANCED, NATURAL LIQUID SURFACTANT/SOAP BASE THAT CAN BE USED FOR A VARIETY OF SOAPY PRODUCTS. YOU CAN MAKE SHOWER GEL, FOAM BATH AND HAND SOAP FROM THE RECIPE PROVIDED BELOW.

MAKES 200 ML

200 ml liquid surfactant base
10 ml boiled and cooled water

1. Mix the liquid surfactant base with the water in a plastic jug. Stir well, and then add the essential oils (see variations below) and mix well.
2. If the mixture becomes too thick, then simply add another 5 ml boiled and cooled water until the desired consistency is acquired.

Variations – add the following essential oils:

Uplifting shower gel: 6 drops peppermint, 12 drops sweet orange and 6 drops basil
Detoxifying shower gel: 6 drops fennel, 6 drops lemongrass, 8 drops grapefruit
Deep forest shower gel: 5 drops lavender, 8 drops cedarwood, 8 drops pine, 4 drops cypress
Floral fantasy shower gel: 8 drops jasmine, 6 drops neroli, 6 drops rose geranium, 3 drops lavender

Soy massage candles

SOY CANDLE WAX IS DERIVED FROM THE SOYA BEAN. SOY WAX IS EXTREMELY NOURISHING FOR THE SKIN AND CAN BE USED TO MOISTURIZE AND TREAT DRY SKIN. THIS RECIPE CONTAINS RELAXING OILS TO HELP YOU UNWIND AND DE-STRESS. USE AFTER YOUR BATH TREATMENT TO REHYDRATE AND MOISTURIZE THE SKIN.

MAKES 3 CANDLES

3 x 15-cm candlewick lengths
   (LX20 thickness)
3 candlewick sustainers
1 pair pliers
silicone glue (available from
   hardware stores)
3 whiskey glass tumblers
500 g soy candle wax
20 g shea butter
10 ml coconut oil
10 ml lavender essential oil
   (1 small bottle)
5 ml neroli essential oil (½ small
   bottle)

1. Prepare the glass tumblers the evening before by pushing the wicks through the candlewick sustainers. Squash the centre of the wick sustainer with a pair of pliers to keep the wick in place.
2. Squeeze a small amount of silicone glue onto the bottom of the glass tumblers, in the centre. Press the smooth side of the wick sustainer onto the glue and allow to set overnight.
3. Heat the soy candle wax, shea butter and coconut oil together in a saucepan over very low heat until completely melted. Stir in the essential oils.
4. Holding the wicks upright, pour the candle wax mixture into the glasses and allow to set.
5. Once the candles have set, trim the wicks using scissors.

How do I use the massage candles? Once the candle is burning and some wax has melted, carefully dip your finger into the melted wax – be careful not to burn your finger on the flame – and use the liquid melted wax to rub into the skin.

Foam bath or shower gels

Bath milk soaks

EGYPTIAN BEAUTY CLEOPATRA USED TO BATH IN MILK TO KEEP HER SKIN SOFT AND SILKY. FEEL LIKE A QUEEN WITH THESE LUXURIOUS MILK SOAK TREATS!

Hydrating rose and patchouli bath milk soak

MAKES 250 ML

200 ml full-cream milk powder
50 ml bicarbonate of soda
25 ml fine sea salt
50 ml dried rose petals (torn into small pieces)
8 drops patchouli essential oil
6 drops rose essential oil
12 drops rose geranium essential oil

1. Place the milk powder, bicarbonate of soda, sea salt and rose petals in a bowl and mix together.
2. Add the essential oils and mix well.
3. Spoon the mixture into a glass or plastic container.

How do I use the milk soak powder? Add a handful of bath milk soak powder to warm bath water for a luxurious bath soak treat.

Orange, neroli and rosemary bath milk soak

THE POWDERED MILK AND BICARBONATE OF SODA SOFTEN THE WATER, WHILE THE ESSENTIAL OILS OF ORANGE, NEROLI AND LAVENDER HAVE SOOTHING AND RELAXING PROPERTIES. DID YOU KNOW THAT NEROLI ESSENTIAL OIL COMES FROM THE FLOWERS OF THE ORANGE TREE?

MAKES 250 ML

200 ml full-cream milk powder
50 ml bicarbonate of soda
50 ml dried rosemary
22 drops sweet orange essential oil
12 drops neroli essential oil
6 drops lavender essential oil

1. Place the milk powder, bicarbonate of soda and dried rosemary leaves in a bowl and mix together.
2. Add the essential oils and mix well.
3. Spoon the mixture into a glass or plastic container.

How do I use the milk soak powder? Add a handful of bath milk soak powder to warm bath water for a luxurious bath soak treat.

Hydrating rose and patchouli bath milk soak

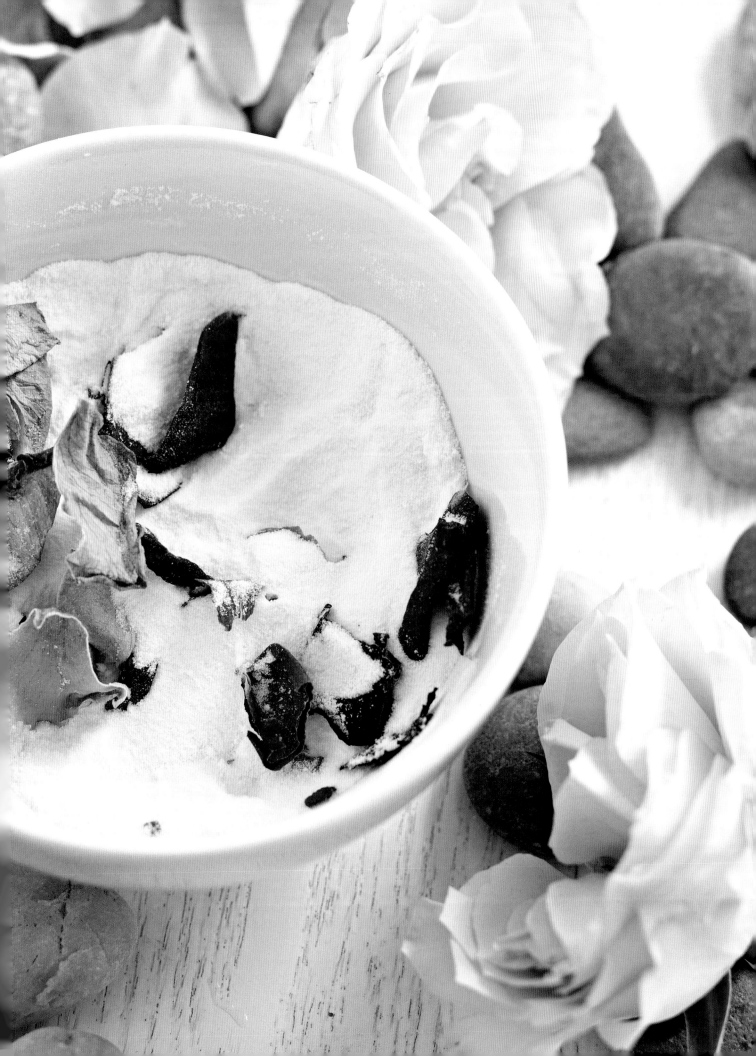

Facial products

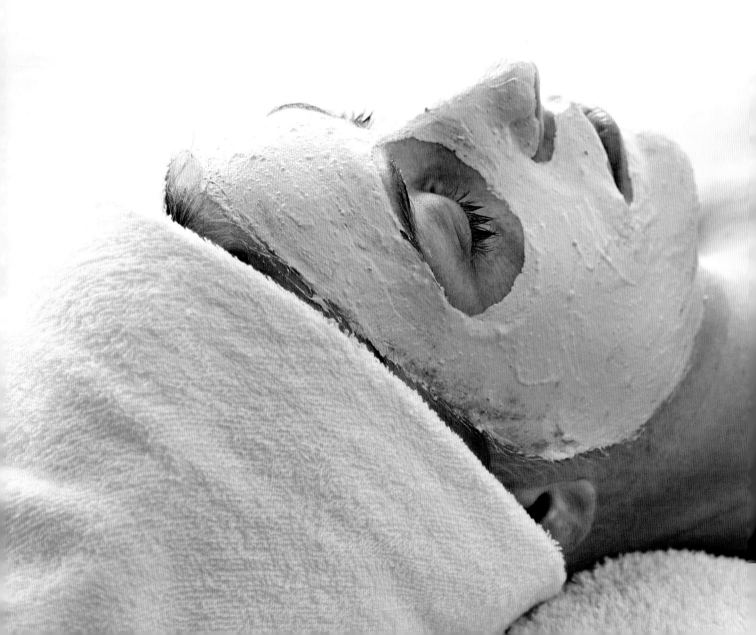

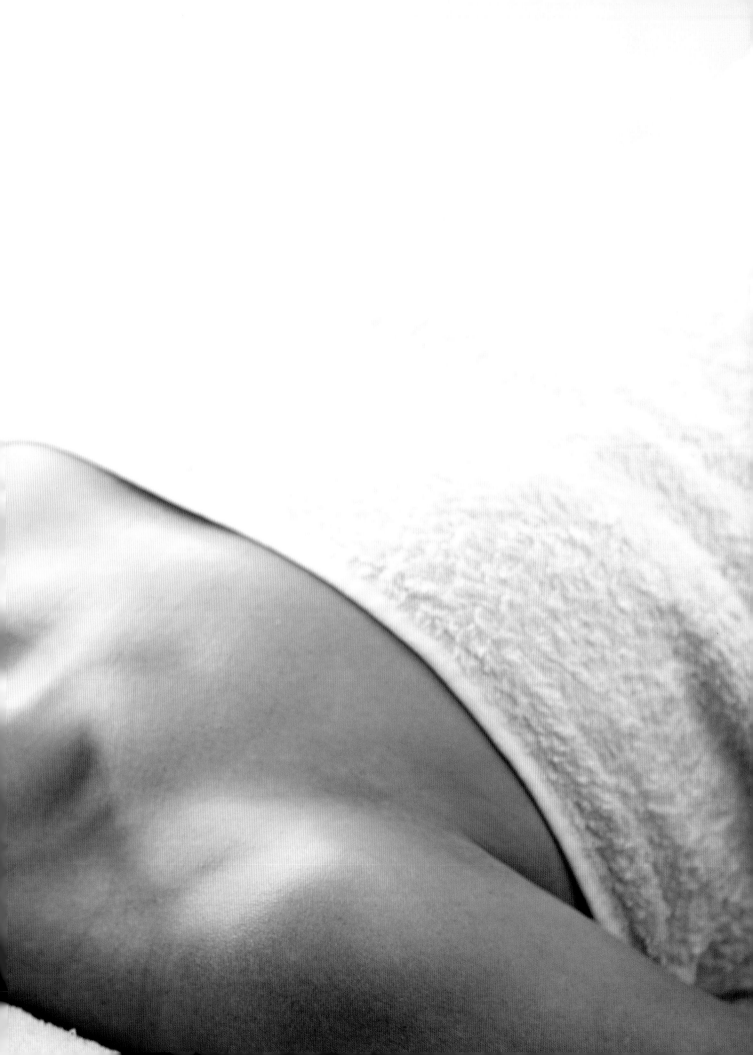

Dark chocolate and mint lip balm

THIS RECIPE INCLUDES REAL DARK CHOCOLATE! I FIRST USED THIS RECIPE FOR A KID'S WORKSHOP AND THE CHILDREN LOVED THE IDEA OF USING REAL CHOCOLATE IN THEIR LIP BALM. A REALLY TASTY TREAT FOR THE LIPS – SWEET CHOCOLATE AND COOL PEPPERMINT – WITH SHEA BUTTER TO HELP PREVENT DRY AND CHAPPED SKIN.

MAKES 2 SMALL JARS

25 ml grapeseed oil
4 g beeswax
10 ml shea butter
6 g dark chocolate
2 drops peppermint essential oil

1. Place the grapeseed oil, beeswax, shea butter and dark chocolate in a saucepan and heat gently until everything is melted.
2. Remove from the heat and add the essential oil. Stir well.
3. Pour carefully into lip balm containers.

How do I use the lip balm? Apply a small amount to the lips as needed.

Lavender milk cleanser

THIS GENTLE CLEANSER MAY BE USED TO REMOVE MAKE-UP AND TO CLEANSE THE FACE.

MAKES 200 ML

150 ml carrier lotion
40 ml carrier cream
10 ml sweet almond oil
3 drops lavender essential oil

1. Mix the carrier lotion, carrier cream and sweet almond oil together with a small whisk until all the ingredients are combined.
2. Add the essential oils and stir well.
3. Pour into a sterilized glass bottle or plastic container.

How do I use the cleanser? Wet your face with warm water and then gently apply the lavender milk cleanser to the face, neck and décolletage. Rinse off with warm water and apply Gentle Rose Water and Witch Hazel Facial Toner (see below) and Revitalizing Face Cream or Balancing Face Cream (see recipes on page 71).

Gentle rose water and witch hazel facial toner

I LIKE TO USE A SPRAY BOTTLE, AND SPRAY THE FACIAL TONER DIRECTLY ONTO THE SKIN. THE SUBTLE ROSE FRAGRANCE IS SO PLEASANT AND THE WITCH HAZEL HAS ASTRINGENT PROPERTIES, WHICH HELPS TO TONE AND REFRESH THE SKIN. I HAVE USED THE WATER FROM THE DISTILLATION PROCESS OF ESSENTIAL OILS, CALLED HYDROSOL/HYDROLAT. EITHER ROSE GERANIUM OR LAVENDER HYDROSOL/HYDROLAT MAY BE USED IN THIS RECIPE.

MAKES 120 ML

100 ml rose geranium or lavender hydrosol/hydrolat
20 ml witch hazel solution
1 drop rose geranium essential oil

1. Pour the hydrolat and witch hazel into a glass or plastic container.
2. Add the essential oil, close the container and shake well.

How do I use the toner? Apply directly to cleansed skin to tone and refresh. Follow with Revitalizing Face Cream or Balancing Face Cream (see recipes on page 71) or Men's After-shave Balm (see page 72).

Lavender milk cleanser and
Gentle rose water and witch hazel facial toner

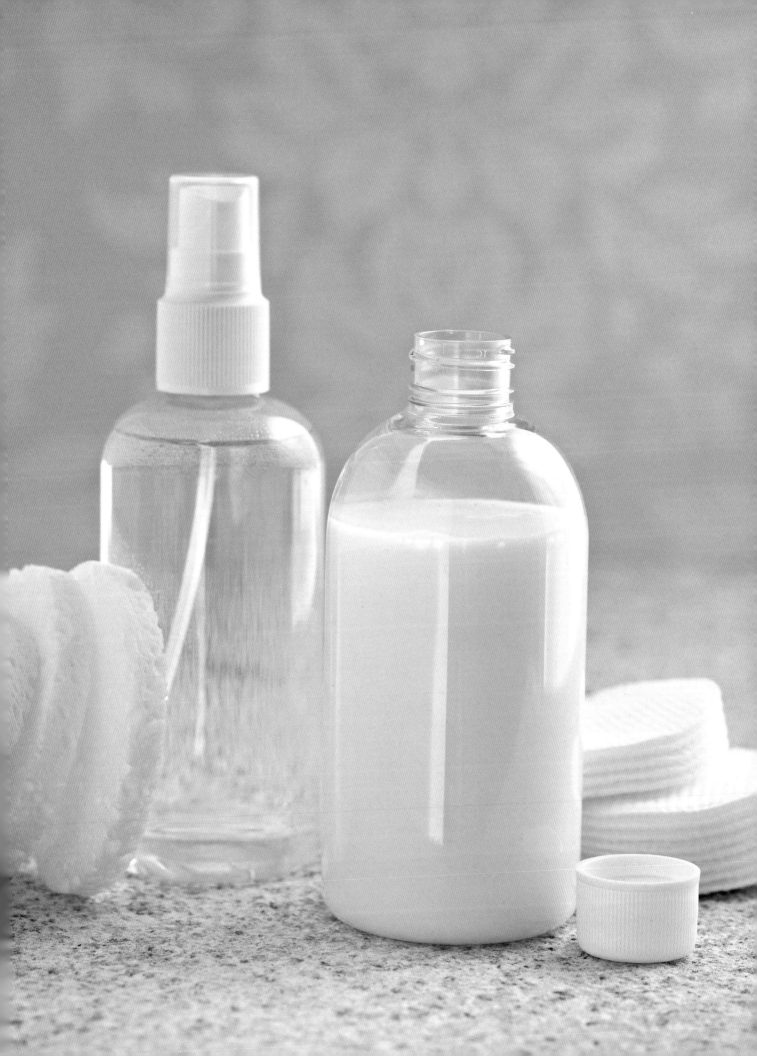

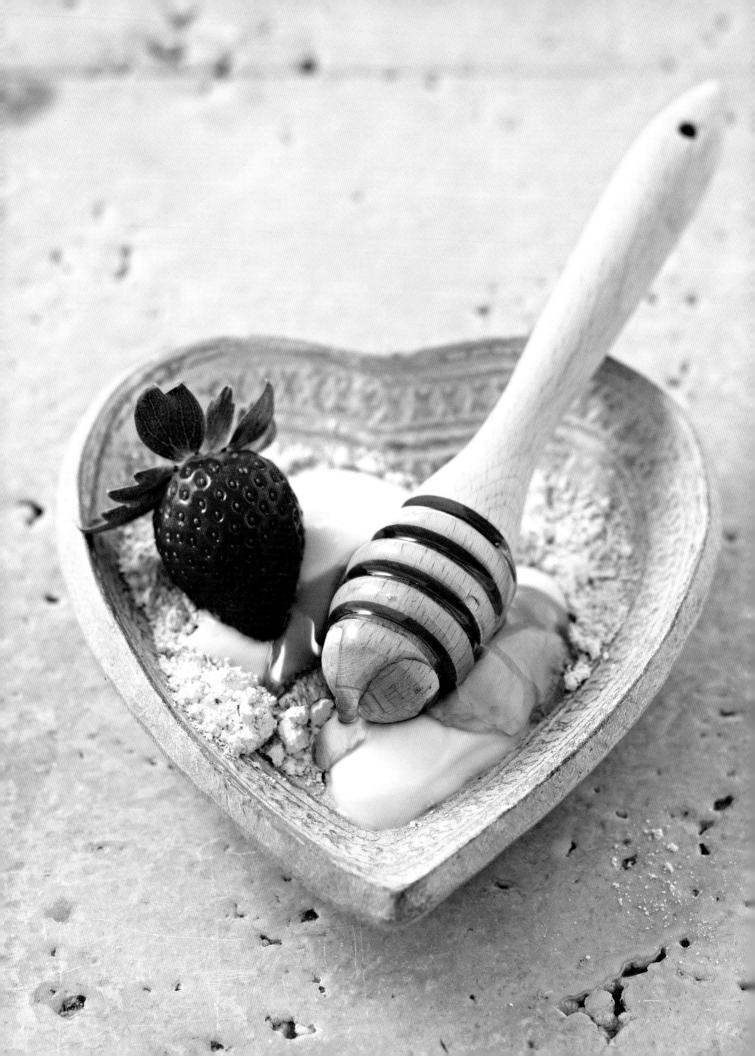

Strawberry vitality mask

STRAWBERRIES ARE HIGH IN VITAMIN C AND ARE GREAT TO GET YOUR SKIN GLOWING
AND EXFOLIATED WITH NATURAL FRUIT ACIDS.

MAKES ENOUGH FOR 1 APPLICATION

1 strawberry
2.5 ml honey
2.5 ml olive oil
15 ml natural plain yoghurt
40 ml kaolin clay powder or bentonite
   clay powder

1. Place all the ingredients in a food processor and whizz together until the clay is smooth and the mask is thick enough to apply to the skin.

How do I use the clay mask?
Apply to cleansed skin and leave for 5–7 minutes. Rinse gently with warm water to remove the mask.

Deep-cleansing and exfoliating kaolin clay mask

KAOLIN CLAY, ALSO KNOWN AS CHINA CLAY, IS AN EXCELLENT NATURAL MINERAL CLAY POWDER THAT IS RICH IN SILICA, MAGNESIUM, SODIUM, IRON AND ZINC. THIS NATURALLY EXFOLIATING MASK TREATMENT IS FOR NORMAL TO OILY SKIN CONDITIONS, WITH THE KAOLIN CLAY BINDING TO DEAD SKIN CELLS AND HELPING TO REMOVE EXCESS OIL. WITCH HAZEL HAS ASTRINGENT PROPERTIES, WHICH MAY HELP TO MINIMIZE LARGE PORES AND CAN BE EFFECTIVE IN THE TREATMENT OF ACNE BY HAVING A SOOTHING EFFECT ON THE SKIN. THIS MASK WILL BE ENOUGH FOR 1 APPLICATION (MAYBE 2), BUT I HAVE KEPT THE QUANTITIES SMALL SO THAT THE MASK CAN BE USED UP IMMEDIATELY. NO PRESERVATIVES MEAN THAT THE PRODUCT MAY SPOIL AND THIS MASK SHOULD BE USED WITHIN A DAY OR TWO. IF THERE IS ANY LEFTOVER MASK, YOU MAY KEEP IT COVERED WITH SOME PLASTIC WRAP AND STORE IT IN THE FRIDGE. ALLOW THE MASK TO RETURN TO ROOM TEMPERATURE BEFORE USING IT.

MAKES ENOUGH FOR 1–2 APPLICATIONS

60 ml kaolin clay powder
15 ml witch hazel solution
15 ml filtered water
1 drop tea tree essential oil

1. Combine all the ingredients in a small bowl and stir until you achieve a smooth consistency. If the mixture is too dry, add a little more witch hazel, and if the mixture is too runny then add a little more clay.

How do I use the clay mask? Apply to cleansed skin and allow to dry (up to 10 minutes). Remove gently with moist cosmetic sponges and rinse with warm water. Use once a week for normal skin, and up to three times a week for acne.

Strawberry vitality mask

Avocado crème mask

DON'T THROW THAT LEFTOVER AVOCADO AWAY – HAUL IT OUT OF THE FRIDGE AND FEED YOUR SKIN! THIS MASK GIVES EXTRA MOISTURE AND OIL TO DRY SKIN CONDITIONS. THE MASK IS BEST USED IMMEDIATELY AS IT DOES NOT KEEP WELL.

MAKES ENOUGH FOR 1 MASK TREATMENT

¼ ripe avocado
5 ml extra virgin olive oil

1. Mash the avocado and add the olive oil. Mix well until the oil is fully incorporated. Place in a food processor and whizz for a few seconds until the mask is smooth and creamy.

How do I use the mask? Apply to cleansed skin and leave for 5 minutes. Fill a basin with warm water (for removing the mask later) and dip your hands into the water. Using very gentle circular movements, massage the mask into your face. Leave the mask on your face for another 5–10 minutes. Remove with warm water.

Tip: Use any leftover mask as a nourishing hand mask.

Egg white protein firming mask

A FIRM FAVOURITE. EGG WHITE IS RICH IN PROTEIN AS WELL AS MINERALS SUCH AS POTASSIUM, SODIUM AND MAGNESIUM. EGG WHITE IS AN ASTRINGENT WHICH, AS IT DRIES ON YOUR SKIN, CAN HELP TO TIGHTEN AND FIRM THE SKIN. USE THIS MASK IMMEDIATELY.

MAKES ENOUGH FOR 1 MASK TREATMENT

1 egg white

1. Whisk the egg white until it is white and foamy.

How do I use the mask?
Apply to cleansed face and décolletage and allow to dry for about 5 minutes (you will feel the firming effect). Rinse with warm water to remove the mask.

Avocado crème mask

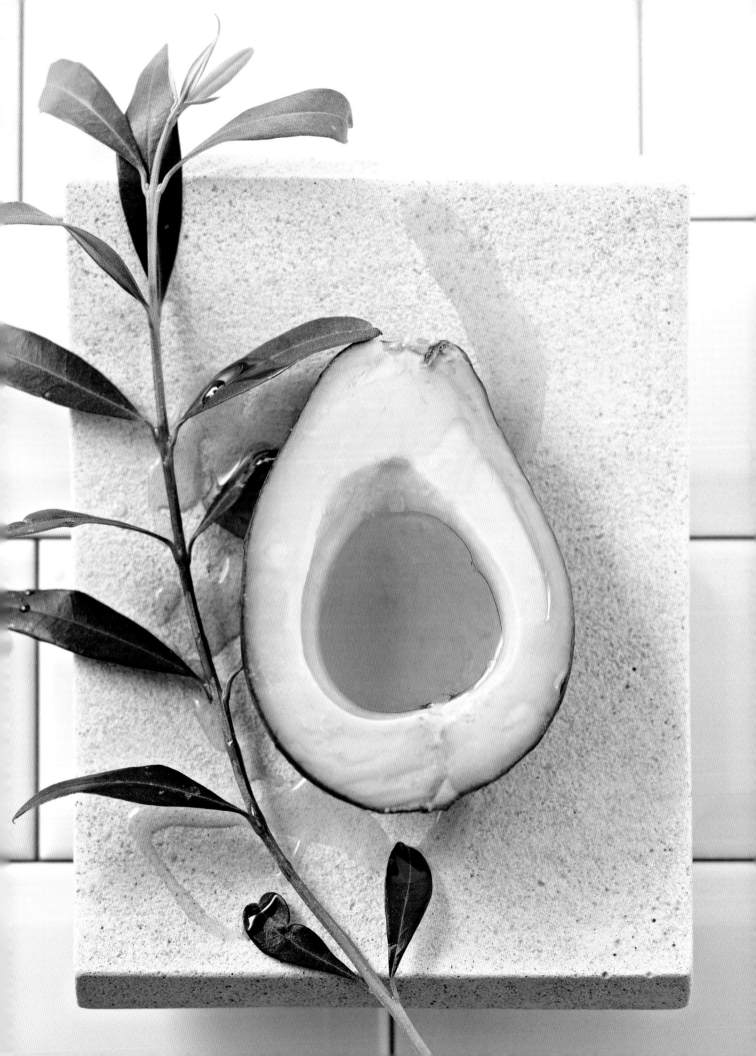

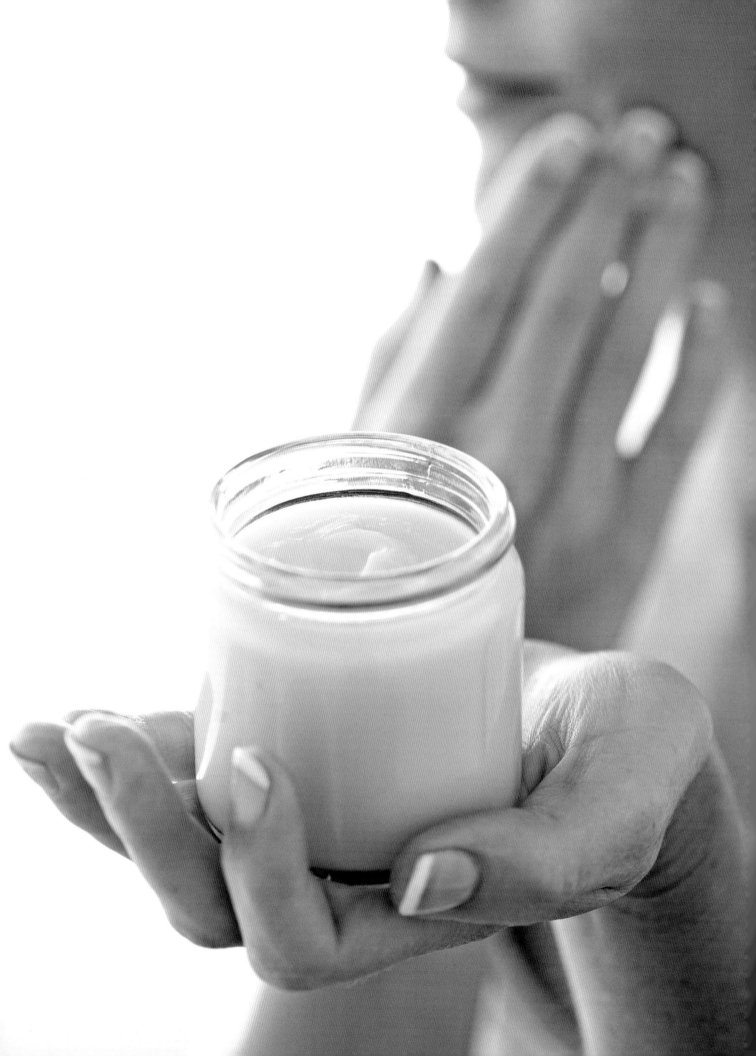

Hydrating treatment mask

THE COMBINATION OF THE WATER-BASED CARRIER GEL AND THE OILS MAKE THIS MASK IDEAL FOR SKIN THAT LACKS MOISTURE AND HYDRATION. IT IS SUITABLE FOR NORMAL, DRY OR COMBINATION SKIN.

MAKES ENOUGH FOR ABOUT 3 APPLICATIONS

10 ml shea butter
10 ml carrier cream
5 ml carrier gel
10 ml sweet almond oil
2 drops neroli essential oil

1. Melt the shea butter in a saucepan over low heat. Once melted, place the saucepan in the fridge (so that the shea butter can solidify again).
2. Mix the carrier cream, carrier gel, sweet almond oil and essential oil together in a bowl.
3. When the shea butter is the consistency of soft butter, remove from the fridge and mix it into the rest of the ingredients. Stir well.
4. Store in a sterilized glass or plastic container.

How do I use the treatment mask? Cleanse the skin and dry gently before applying this mask. Apply about 7.5 ml to the face and décolletage (you can also include the lips and area surrounding the lips and around the eyes). Allow the mask to work into the skin for 10–15 minutes and then rinse with lukewarm water to remove. Apply Gentle Rose Water and Witch Hazel Facial Toner (see page 64), Revitalizing or Balancing Face Cream (see below) or Men's After-shave Balm (see page 72).

Balancing face cream

WITH JOJOBA OIL (RENOWNED FOR ITS COMPATIBILITY WITH THE SKIN'S OWN SEBUM) AND ANTI-MICROBIAL AND SKIN-SOOTHING ESSENTIAL OILS OF TEA TREE, SANDALWOOD AND ROSE GERANIUM.

MAKES 50 ML

50 ml carrier cream
5 ml jojoba oil
1 drop rose geranium essential oil
2 drops sandalwood essential oil
2 drops tea tree essential oil

1. Place the carrier cream and jojoba oil in a bowl and mix well. Add the essential oils and mix through.
2. Spoon the cream into a sterilized glass or plastic jar.

Revitalizing face cream

REGENERATING AND REVITALIZING FOR THE SKIN – WITH ADDED CARROT OIL, WHICH IS RICH IN ANTIOXIDANTS, AND NEROLI OIL.

MAKES 50 ML

50 ml carrier cream
2.5 ml carrot oil
2 drops neroli essential oil
1 drop rose essential oil

1. Place the carrier cream and carrot oil in a bowl and mix well. Add the essential oils and mix through.
2. Spoon the cream into a sterilized glass or plastic jar.

Revitalizing face cream

Men's after-shave balm

MASCULINE SCENTS OF SANDALWOOD AND CEDARWOOD ESSENTIAL OILS MAKE THIS A POPULAR BLEND FOR
A SOOTHING AFTER-SHAVE BALM. LAVENDER ESSENTIAL OIL ALSO HELPS TO CALM SKIN IRRITATION AND
IS USED FOR ITS REGENERATING PROPERTIES.

MAKES 50 ML

50 ml carrier cream
5 ml jojoba oil
2 drops sandalwood essential oil
2 drops cedarwood essential oil
1 drop lavender essential oil

1. Place the carrier cream and jojoba oil in a bowl and mix well. Add the essential oils and mix through.
2. Spoon the cream into a sterilized glass or plastic jar.

How do I use the after-shave balm? Apply the balm to the skin immediately after shaving.

Soothing eye cream

WATER-BASED GEL, SWEET ALMOND OIL AND FRANKINCENSE ARE COMBINED TO CREATE A SOOTHING EYE GEL –
USEFUL FOR HELPING TO REVITALIZE THE SKIN SURROUNDING THE EYES.

MAKES 35 ML

30 ml carrier gel
5 ml sweet almond oil
**1 drop frankincense essential oil (or
  1 drop lavender essential oil if you
  don't have frankincense)**

1. Place the carrier gel and sweet almond oil together in a bowl and mix well.
2. Add the essential oil and mix through.
3. Spoon into a small lip balm-sized container.

How do I use the eye cream? Apply a very small amount to the area underneath the eye before applying your day cream.

Men's after-shave balm

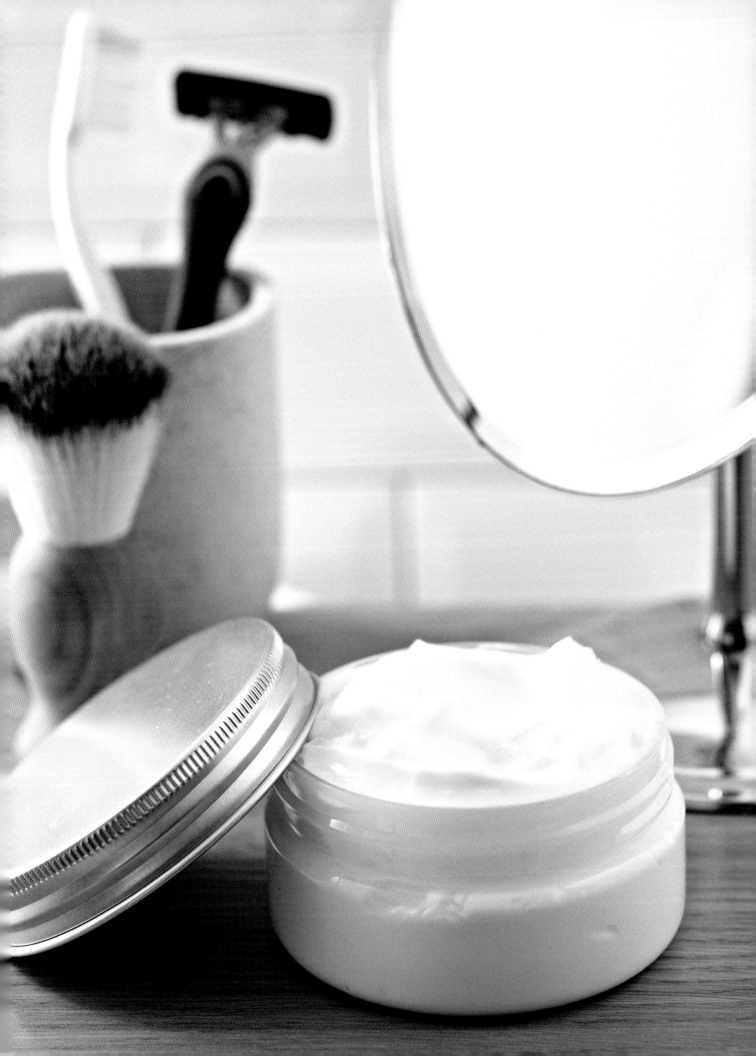

Products for
pregnancy and childbirth

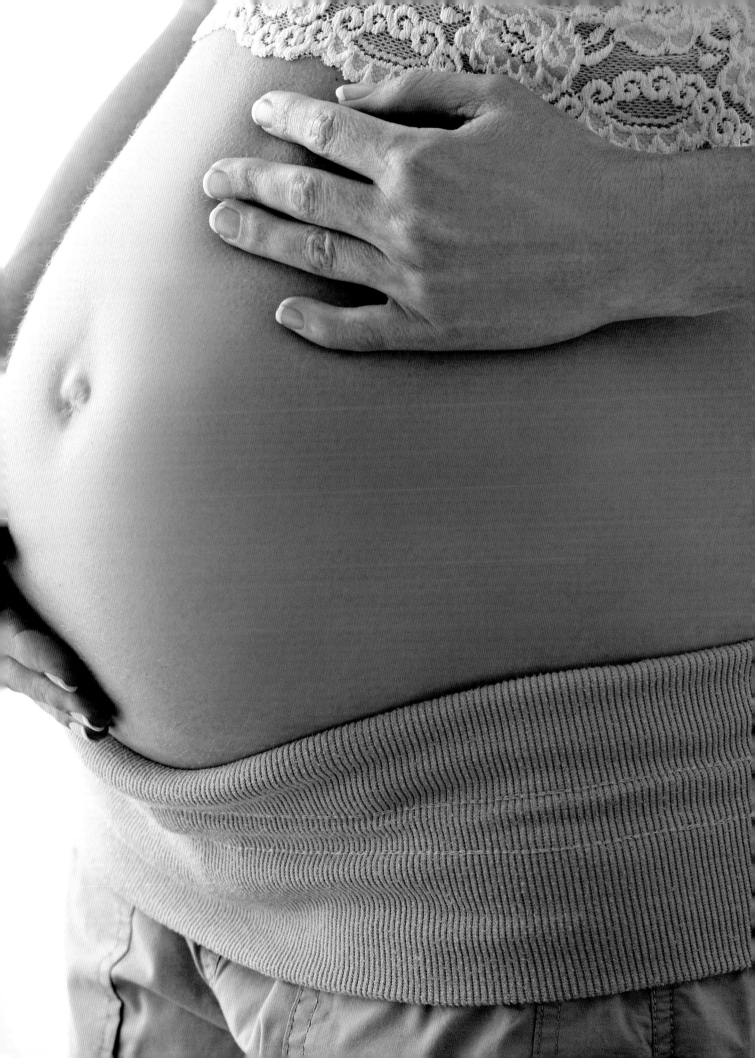

Stretch mark oil

THIS BODY OIL IS SCENTED WITH ORANGE FLOWER (NEROLI) ESSENTIAL OIL AND ENHANCED WITH CARROT AND ROSE HIP OILS TO INCREASE SKIN CELL TURNOVER AND THEREFORE HELP TO PREVENT STRETCH MARKS AND DRY SKIN.

MAKES 100 ML

85 ml sweet almond oil
10 ml rose hip oil
2 drops carrot oil
2 drops neroli essential oil
2 drops rosewood essential oil

1. Mix the sweet almond, rose hip and carrot oils together in a bottle.
2. Add the essential oils and shake well.

How do I use the oil? Add a little oil to bath water or apply directly onto dry skin to relieve itchiness and dryness.

Hydrating all-over body cream

YOUR SKIN MAY NEED EXTRA MOISTURE DURING PREGNANCY AND, AS THE SKIN STRETCHES, IT CAN BECOME DRY AND ITCHY. THIS RECIPE IS ENRICHED WITH OLIVE OIL TO NOURISH THE SKIN, AND ROSE HIP TO INCREASE ELASTICITY. THE PRODUCT IS GENTLE ENOUGH FOR YOUR FACE, BODY AND FEET.

MAKES 250 ML

250 ml thickened carrier cream
10 ml olive oil
5 ml sweet almond oil
10 ml rose hip oil
4 drops neroli essential oil
1 drop petitgrain essential oil
2 drops sweet orange essential oil

1. Mix all the ingredients together.

Did you know? The essential oils used in this recipe are all produced from the orange tree – orange (from the fruit), petitgrain (from the twigs and leaves) and neroli (from the blossoms). These essential oils create perfect synergy for relaxation and help to keep your skin looking good too!

Relaxing bath oil (for pregnancy)

USE THIS BATH OIL TO EASE YOUR TIRED MUSCLES DURING PREGNANCY. ESSENTIAL OILS OF NEROLI, MANDARIN AND YLANG YLANG ARE GENTLE AND CALMING.

MAKES 100 ML

100 ml grapeseed oil
5 drops neroli essential oil
3 drops mandarin essential oil
2 drops ylang ylang essential oil

1. Mix the grapeseed oil and essential oils together in a bottle.
2. Shake well to disperse the essential oils.

How do I use the bath oil? Add a little oil to your bath water for a relaxing bath soak treatment.

Hydrating all-over body cream

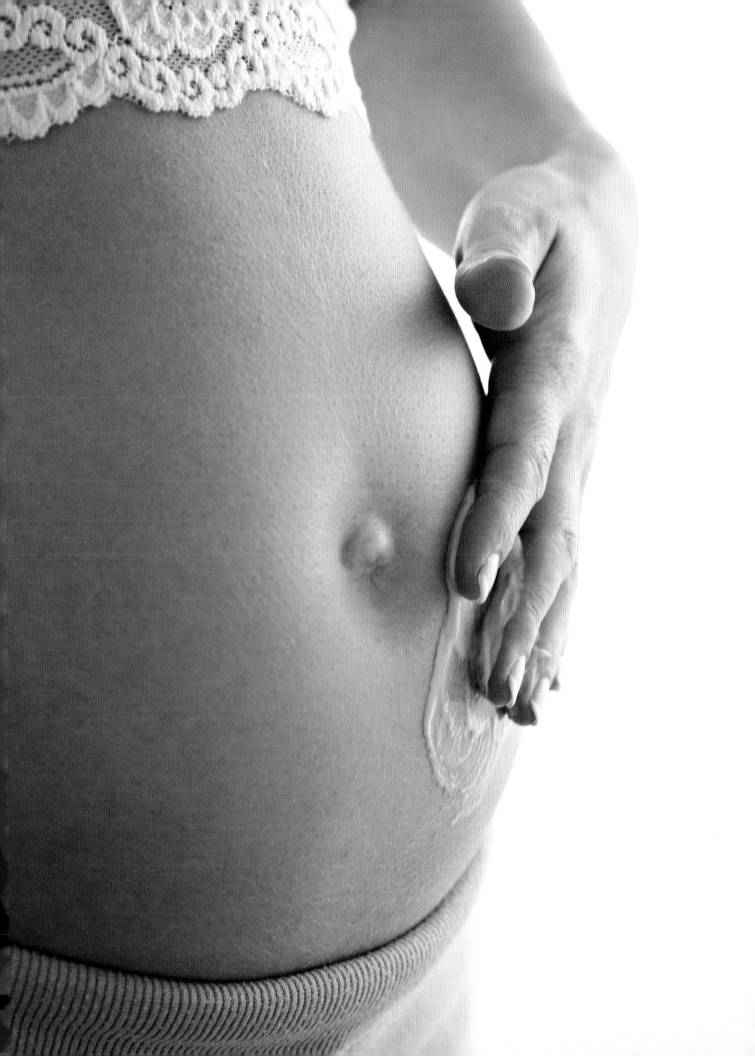

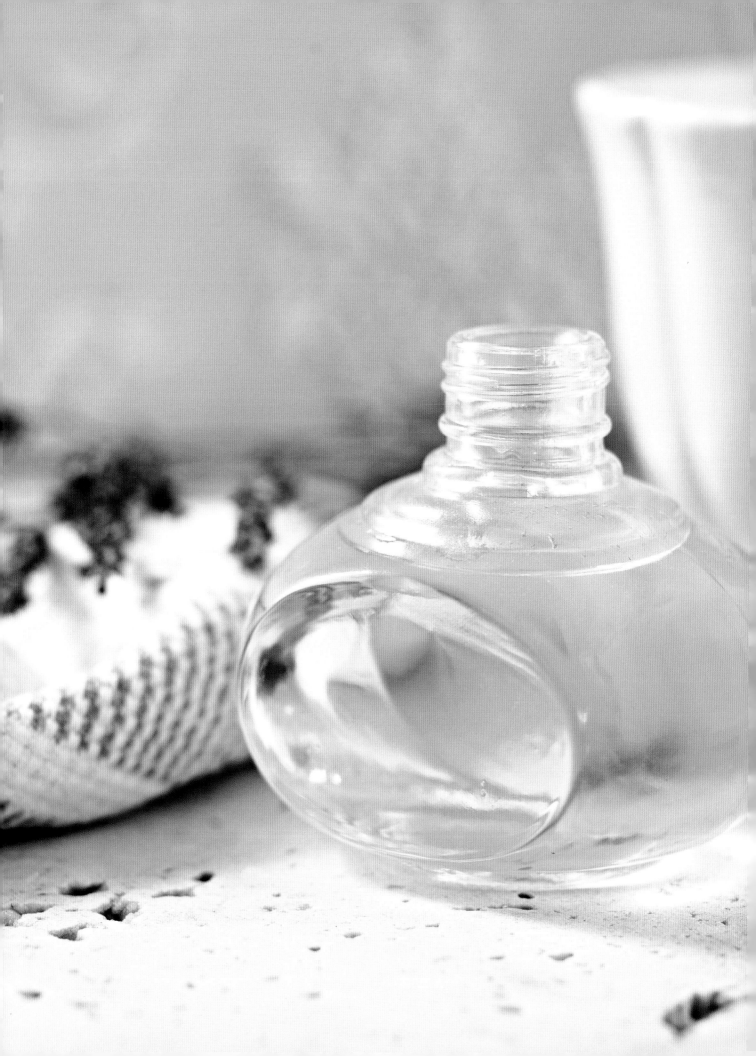

Bath/massage oil for labour and childbirth

A RELAXING, YET POWERFUL AROMATHERAPY BLEND OF ESSENTIAL OILS MAKE THIS OIL AN IDEAL CHOICE
FOR MASSAGE DURING CHILDBIRTH. THE LOWER BACK AND HIPS ARE OFTEN TENSE AND TIRED, AND THESE
ESSENTIAL OILS ALSO HAVE ANTI-INFLAMMATORY AND PAIN-RELIEVING PROPERTIES. THE LAVENDER
AND JASMINE ESSENTIAL OILS CAN HELP TO PROMOTE CONTRACTIONS AS WELL AS DULL UTERINE PAIN,
WHILE THE CLARY SAGE ESSENTIAL OIL CAN HELP TO RELIEVE TENSION AND BRING ON LABOUR.

Note: This particular massage/bath oil should only be used during
labour and childbirth and is contra-indicated for use before your baby has reached full-term.

MAKES 100 ML

100 ml grapeseed oil
12 drops jasmine essential oil
10 drops lavender essential oil
8 drops clary sage essential oil

1. Mix the grapeseed oil and essential oils together in a bottle.
2. Shake well to disperse the essential oils.

How do I use the oil? Use as a massage oil to help relieve tired and tense
muscles of the lower back and abdomen during labour. During a water birth,
add 5–10 ml oil to the bath water.

Perineum oil (preparation for natural birth)

THIS OIL CAN BE APPLIED AND GENTLY MASSAGED INTO THE PERINEUM DAILY DURING THE LAST TRIMESTER TO HELP
STRENGTHEN AND CREATE ELASTICITY TO FACILITATE NATURAL CHILDBIRTH.

Note: Use only during the third trimester.

MAKES 100 ML

100 ml sweet almond oil
3 drops organic rose essential oil

1. Place the sweet almond oil and essential oil together in a container.
2. Shake well to disperse the essential oil.

How do I use the oil? Massage the perineum with a little oil at least twice a day
to help strengthen the area in preparation for natural childbirth.

Bath/massage oil for labour and childbirth

Healing salt sitz bath

SEA SALT AND ESSENTIAL OILS PROVIDE ANTI-BACTERIAL PROPERTIES AND HELP TO FACILITATE A SPEEDY RECOVERY AFTER NATURAL CHILDBIRTH. TAKE FREQUENT HEALING SALT BATHS DURING THE DAY/NIGHT TO HELP SOOTHE AND EASE PAIN AND INFLAMMATION.

MAKES ENOUGH FOR 6–8 BATHS

1 kg sea salt
4 drops lavender essential oil
4 drops tea tree essential oil

1. Add salt and essential oils together and mix well.

How do I use the salts? Add about 4 handfuls of aromatherapy sea salt to a shallow, warm bath to help soothe and heal the skin.

Calming and healing tea tree and witch hazel post-birth treatment

KEEP THIS HEALING LIQUID MIXTURE IN YOUR BATHROOM CABINET IN A STERILIZED, SEALED CONTAINER AND USE FREQUENTLY TO HELP EASE, SOOTHE AND RELIEVE DISCOMFORT OF THE PERINEUM. WITCH HAZEL HAS ANTI-INFLAMMATORY AND HEALING PROPERTIES, AND THE TEA TREE OIL IS ADDED TO HELP WITH THE HEALING PROCESS.

MAKES 500 ML

200 ml witch hazel solution
300 ml filtered water
3 drops tea tree essential oil
3 drops lavender essential oil

1. Pour all the ingredients into a sterilized 500 ml plastic bottle and shake well to disperse the essential oils.

How do I use the treatment? Keep the mixture in the bathroom near the toilet so that you can use it as a rinse every time you visit the bathroom. It can also be used as a vaginal douche to encourage healing and prevent infection.

Healing salt sitz bath and
Calming and healing tea tree and witch hazel post-birth treatment

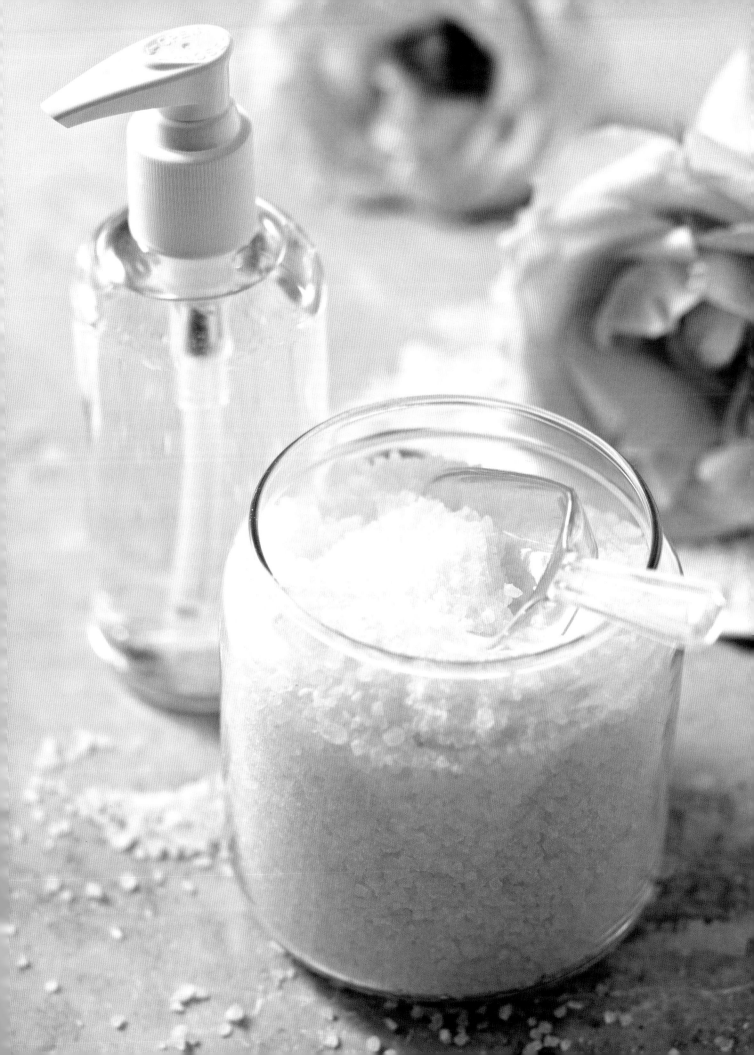

Products for babies

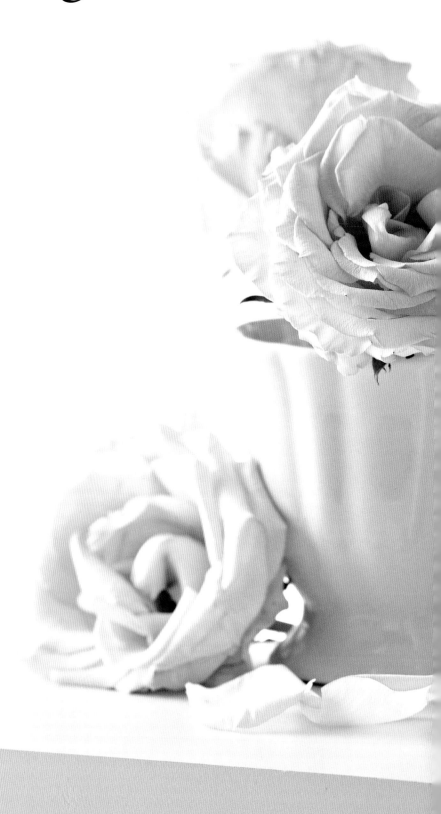

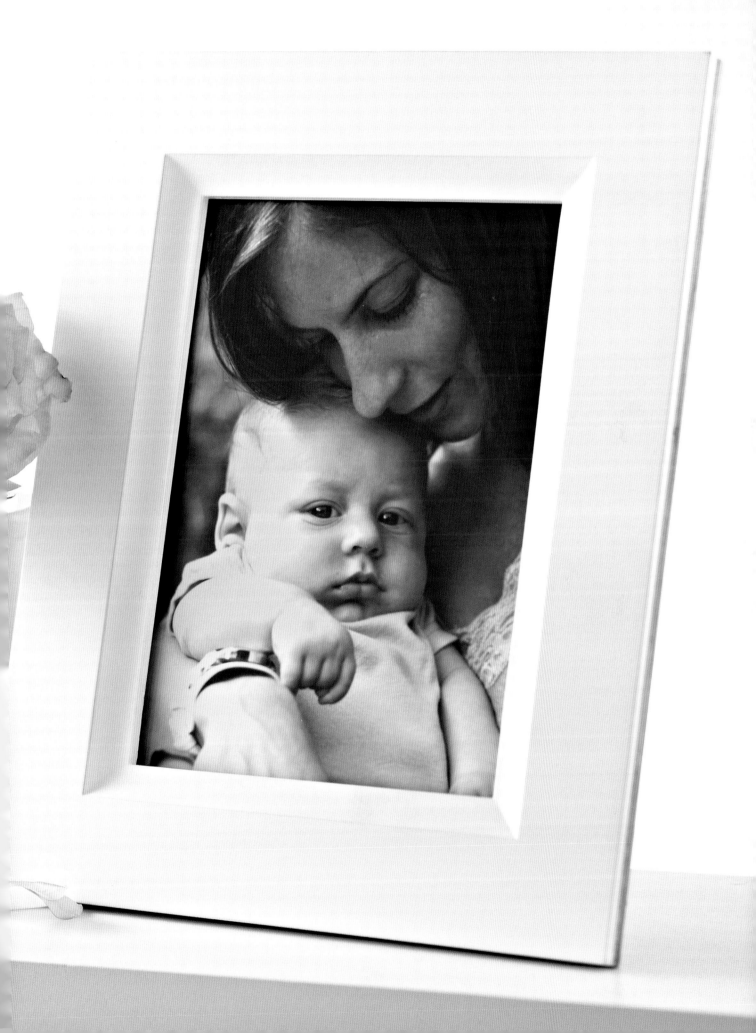

I PREFER TO USE THE BEST QUALITY, 100% CERTIFIED ORGANIC ESSENTIAL OILS IN MY BABY PRODUCTS BECAUSE
I KNOW THAT THEY ARE FREE OF ANY POSSIBLE PESTICIDE RESIDUE. YOU CAN PURCHASE ORGANIC ESSENTIAL OILS
FROM YOUR LOCAL HEALTH SHOP OR PHARMACY.

Gentle baby wash

MAKES 200 ML

180 ml unfragranced surfactant base
(liquid soap base)
20 ml boiling water
10 ml sweet almond oil
2 drops organic lavender essential oil
2 drops organic mandarin essential oil

1. Mix the surfactant base, boiling water and sweet almond oil together in a plastic or glass jug. Stir together. Add the essential oils and mix again until the essential oils are mixed through.
2. Pour into a sterilized plastic or glass container.

How do I use the baby wash? Use a small amount of gentle baby wash per bath (2.5 ml will be more than enough). Alternatively, add 2.5 ml to running bath water to create an aromatherapy foam bath.

Lavender and chamomile natural baby powder

COMMERCIAL BABY POWDERS CONTAIN TALCUM POWDER, WHICH IS CLOSELY RELATED TO THE CARCINOGEN, ASBESTOS. STUDIES
HAVE SHOWN THAT TINY PARTICLES (EASILY INHALED BY INFANTS) CAN BECOME IMBEDDED IN THE LUNGS AND RESEARCH HAS
ALSO SHOWN A LINK BETWEEN PATIENTS WHO FREQUENTLY USE TALCUM POWDER ON THE GENITALIA AND OVARIAN CANCER.
USING COMMERCIAL TALCUM POWDER IS UNNECESSARY AND COULD POTENTIALLY BE A HEALTH RISK FOR INFANTS.
THIS NATURAL BABY POWDER USES MOSTLY CORNFLOUR AND IS A HEALTHIER ALTERNATIVE.

MAKES 125 ML

25 ml kaolin clay powder
5 ml rice flour
100 ml cornflour
3 drops organic lavender essential oil
2 drops organic rose geranium
essential oil
1 drop organic Roman chamomile
essential oil

1. Mix the kaolin clay, rice flour and cornflour together in a bowl. Add the essential oils and mix well.
2. Sift the mixture to ensure that all the essential oils are dispersed throughout the powder.
3. Spoon into a sterilized plastic or glass container.

> *Tip:* Use this natural baby powder to keep baby's skin dry and to prevent excess moisture from causing skin irritation.
> I found it particularly useful when my son was cutting his first teeth. Teething can cause a lot of excess saliva
> and the skin on the neck and chest can be constantly damp.

Lavender and chamomile natural baby powder

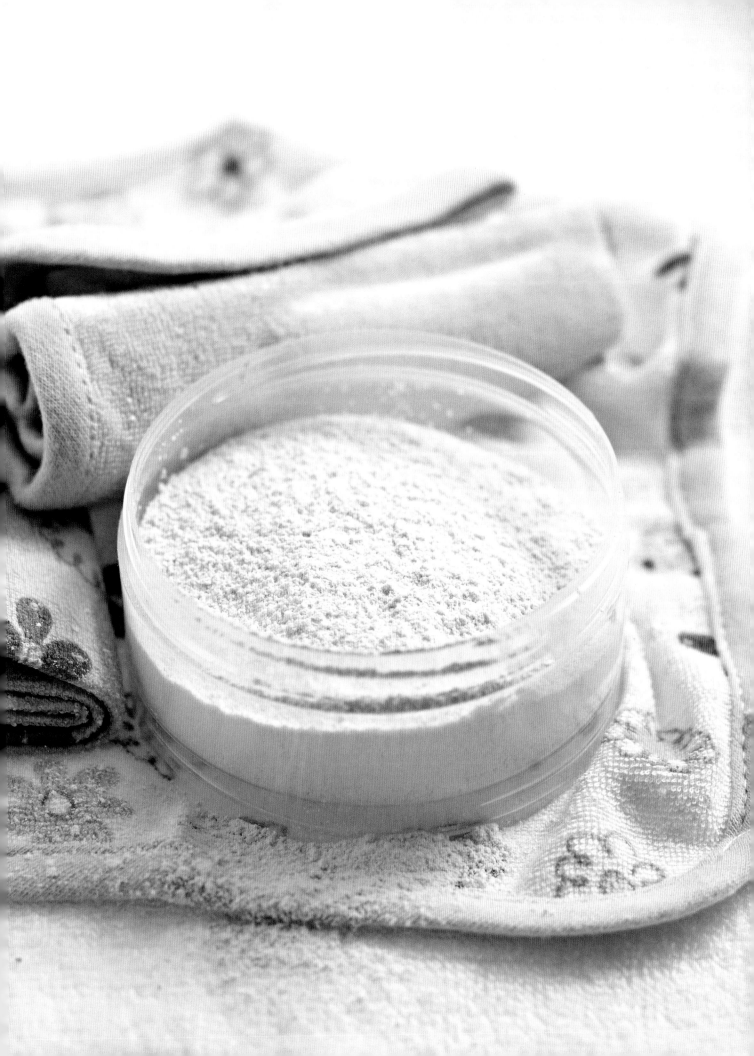

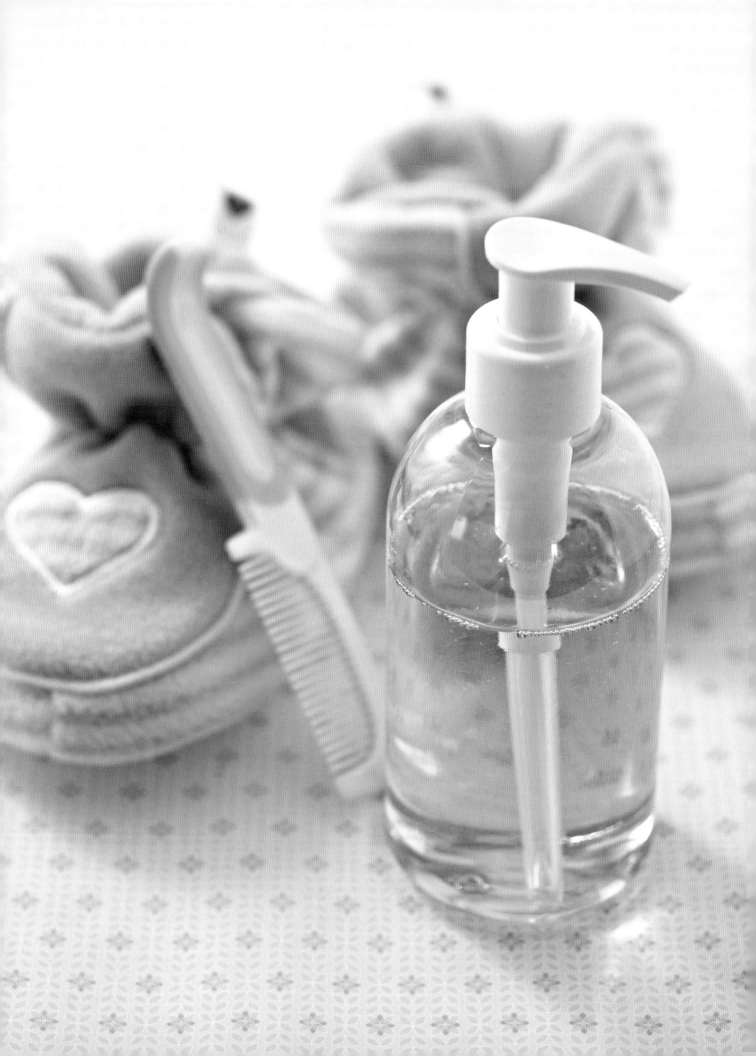

Treatment oil for cradle cap

CRADLE CAP IS A FUNGAL INFECTION THAT MOST BABIES GET AT ONE TIME OR ANOTHER. THIS TREATMENT OIL CAN HELP LOOSEN ANY DEAD SKIN AND THE TEA TREE AND GERANIUM ESSENTIAL OILS HAVE ANTI-FUNGAL PROPERTIES.

MAKES 100 ML

50 ml olive oil
50 ml neem oil
1 drop organic tea tree essential oil
1 drop organic rose geranium
   essential oil

1. Mix all the ingredients together in a sterilized plastic or glass container and shake well.

How do I use the treatment oil? Apply about 2.5 ml oil to the baby's scalp and massage very gently into the hair. Be very careful to use gentle movements as the fontanelle (bones of the skull) has not yet closed properly on newborn babies. Leave the oil on for a few hours and then comb very gently through the hair. Wash the hair with Baby Soap Bar with Lavender, Rose Geranium and Calendula (see page 123) or Gentle Baby Wash (see page 84).

Newborn baby oil

IT IS BEST TO USE PLAIN GRAPESEED OIL FOR NEWBORNS. INTRODUCE ESSENTIAL OILS IN MASSAGE FROM 4 WEEKS ONWARDS.

MAKES 100 ML

100 ml grapeseed oil

How do I use the oil? Gentle massage is advised – it should be more like an application of the product than a massage – as newborn babies are very sensitive.

Did you know? In India, newborn babies are massaged daily with olive oil to help strengthen their limbs.

Treatment oil for cradle cap

Sleepy baby massage oil

THE GRAPESEED OIL WILL HELP TO KEEP THE SKIN SOFT AND MOISTURIZED, WHILE THE LAVENDER AND CHAMOMILE ESSENTIAL OILS CAN HELP TO PROMOTE RELAXATION AND INDUCE SLEEP.

MAKES 100 ML

100 ml grapeseed oil

2 drops organic lavender essential oil

1 drop organic Roman chamomile
    essential oil

1. Mix the grapeseed and essential oils together in a container.
2. Shake well to disperse the essential oils.

How do I use the massage oil? Apply about 2.5 ml oil to baby's skin after a bath.

Variations – to 100 ml grapeseed oil, add the following essential oils:

Calming baby massage oil: 2 drops organic lavender, 2 drops organic mandarin

Sensitive baby massage oil: 1 drop organic lavender

Soothing baby bum cream for nappy rash

THE ZINC OXIDE AND LAVENDER ESSENTIAL OIL HELP TO HEAL THE SKIN AND ARE INDICATED FOR USE ON RASHES AND IRRITATION. BEESWAX AND CASTOR OIL HELP TO FORM A NATURAL BARRIER ON THE SKIN.

MAKES 125 ML

120 ml castor oil

18 g beeswax

25 ml grapeseed oil

15 ml zinc oxide powder

6 drops organic lavender essential oil

1. Place the castor oil, beeswax and grapeseed oil in a saucepan and heat gently over low heat until the beeswax has melted.
2. Remove from the heat and add the zinc oxide powder.
3. Allow to cool slightly and then add the essential oil and mix together.
4. Stir every 5 minutes while cooling so that the zinc oxide is properly emulsified into the mixture.
5. If the mixture starts setting too quickly for you to pour into your containers, heat again very gently just to allow a thick pouring consistency.

How do I use the cream? Apply to areas of nappy rash to soothe the skin and help it heal. Apply to skin as a preventative measure to help create a slight barrier between the nappy and the skin.

Soothing baby bum cream for nappy rash

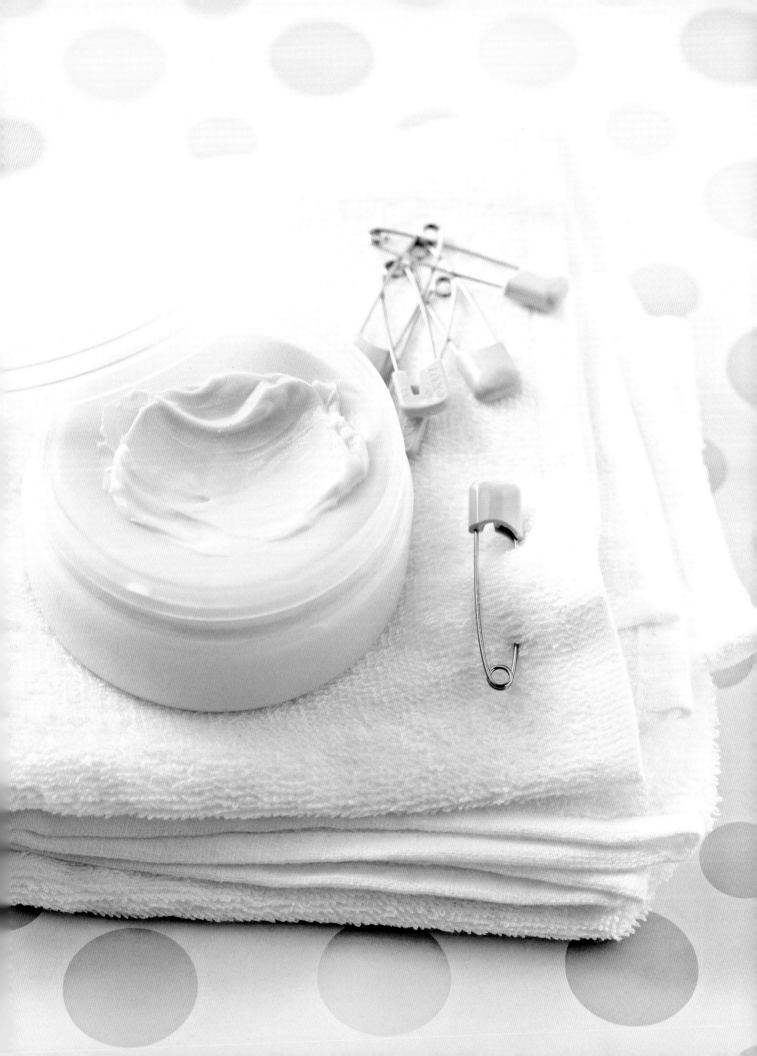

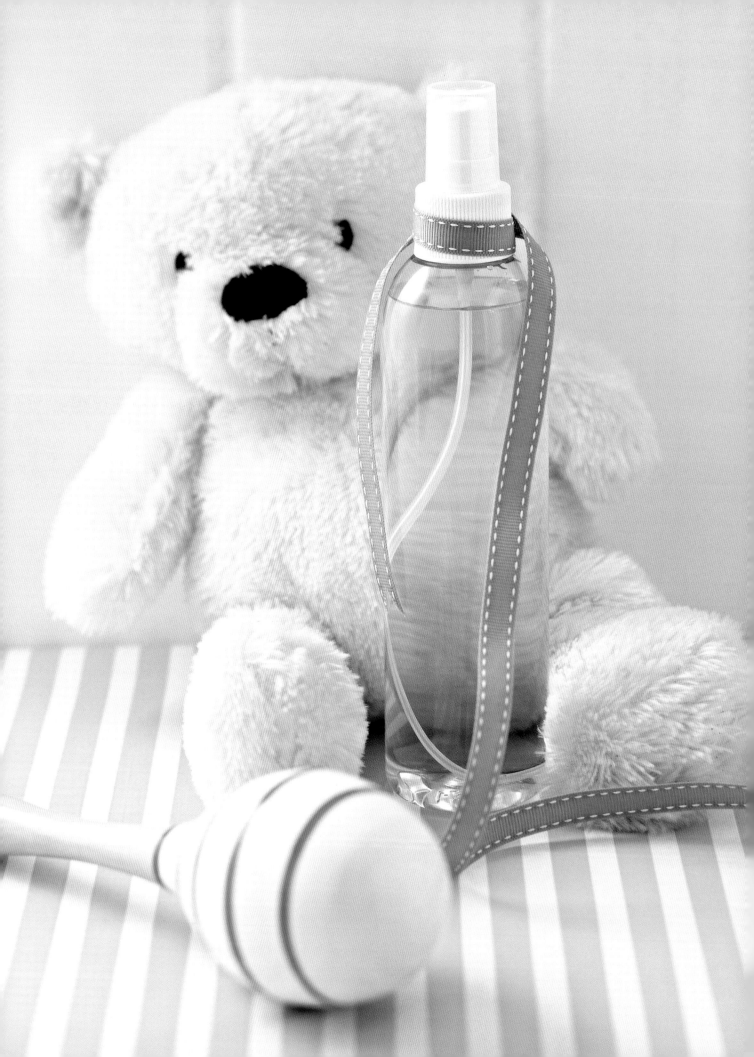

Happy baby aroma room spray

A CALMING AND GENTLE FRAGRANCE FOR KEEPING BABY'S ROOM SMELLING CLEAN AND FRESH! IT CAN ALSO BE SPRAYED ONTO FABRICS AS A REFRESHER.

MAKES 200 ML

200 ml filtered water
6 drops organic lavender essential oil
1 drop organic Roman chamomile
   essential oil

1. Pour the water and essential oils together in a sterilized plastic spray bottle.
2. Shake well to disperse the essential oils.

How do I use the spray? Spray a little in the baby's bedroom as a natural air freshener.

Breathe-easy room spray

SPRAY THIS AROMATIC NATURAL AIR FRESHENER INTO BABY'S ROOM WHEN YOUR BABY IS SUFFERING FROM A BLOCKED NOSE OR COLDS AND FLU. EUCALYPTUS ESSENTIAL OIL IS OFTEN INCLUDED IN ALTERNATIVE MEDICINES TO HELP BOOST THE IMMUNE SYSTEM, AND SANDALWOOD ESSENTIAL OIL CAN HELP TO EASE RESPIRATORY INFECTIONS.

MAKES 200 ML

200 ml filtered water
8 drops organic eucalyptus essential oil
4 drops organic sandalwood
   essential oil

1. Pour the water and essential oils together in a sterilized plastic spray bottle.
2. Shake well to disperse the essential oils.

How do I use the spray? Use as an air freshener. The essential oils are anti-bacterial and make a powerful disinfectant spray.

Helpful hints: Beneficial essential oils for the humidifier

Use 4 drops (in total) of essential oil of your choice. The humidifier helps to keep the air moist and can be a great help for wheezy or chesty coughs. Remember to change the water in the humidifier daily.

Eucalyptus essential oil: expectorant, helps to clear congestion
Tea tree essential oil: anti-microbial, disinfectant
Lavender essential oil: sedative, calming and relaxing

Happy baby aroma room spray

Products for kids

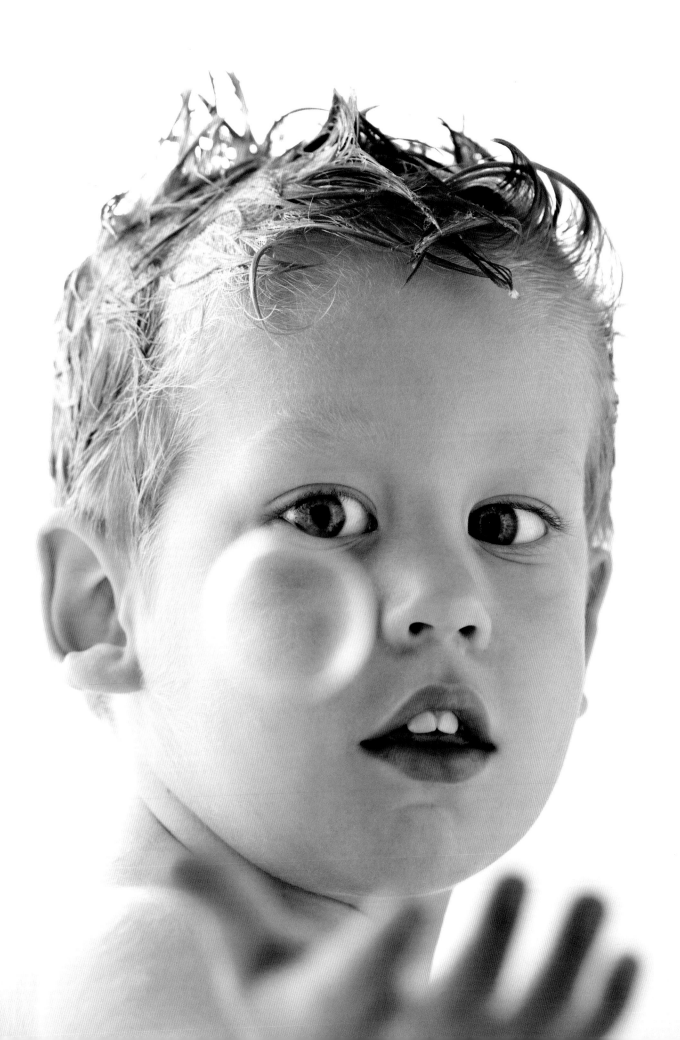

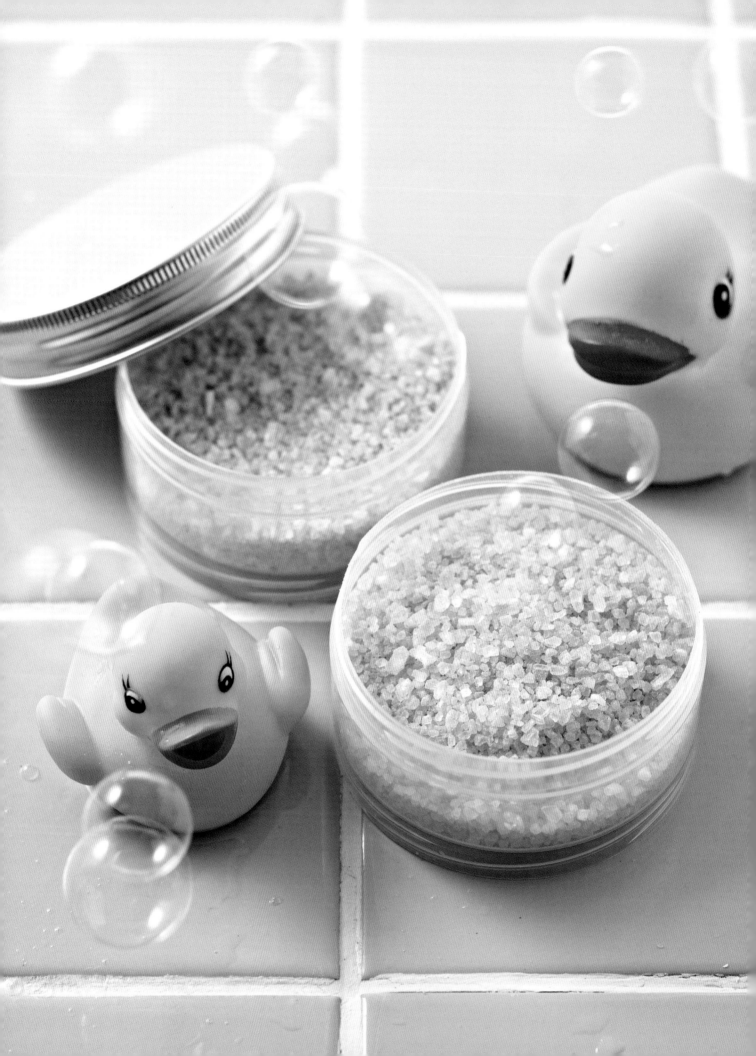

Crazy colour bath salts

KIDS WILL LOVE BATH TIME WITH THESE BATH SALTS. I USE NATURAL COLOURS FROM HERBAL SUPPLEMENTS AND SPICES, BUT YOU CAN USE A DASH OF FOOD COLOURING – USE A VERY SMALL AMOUNT AS SYNTHETIC COLOURING IS VERY CONCENTRATED.

Groovy green bath salts

MAKES 250 ML

250 ml sea salt

2.5 ml spirulina or wheatgrass/barley grass powder (from health shops) OR 0.5 ml green liquid food colouring

5 drops neroli essential oil

5 drops lavender essential oil

3 drops tea tree essential oil

1. Mix the sea salt and colouring together until the colour is evenly distributed.
2. Add the essential oils and mix well.
3. Spoon into sterilized plastic or glass containers.

How do I use the bath salts? Add a handful to the bath and disperse in the water. Agitate the water to dissolve the salt.

Tip: If using spirulina/barley or wheatgrass powder, you will notice that the green colour powder may separate to the bottom of the container – simply shake well before use, and the groovy green colour will return to normal!

Sunshine yellow bath salts

THESE YELLOW BATH SALTS ARE MADE WITH NATURAL COLOUR FROM TURMERIC. UPLIFTING AND SOOTHING ESSENTIAL OILS OF ORANGE, MANDARIN AND ROMAN CHAMOMILE HELP TO CREATE BALANCE AND HARMONY WITHOUT BEING TOO STIMULATING.

MAKES 250 ML

250 ml sea salt

1 ml turmeric

5 drops orange essential oil

5 drops mandarin essential oil

2 drops Roman chamomile essential oil

1. Mix the sea salt and spice together until the colour is evenly distributed.
2. Add the essential oils and mix well.
3. Spoon into sterilized plastic or glass containers.

How do I use the bath salts? Add a handful to the bath and disperse in the water. Agitate the water to dissolve the salt.

Sleeping Beauty bath salts

IN THIS MIXTURE I HAVE USED PINK HIMALAYAN SALT, WHICH HAS CLEANSING AND HEALING PROPERTIES. LAVENDER AND YLANG YLANG HAVE A SOFT FLORAL AROMA AS WELL AS RELAXING, CALMING EFFECTS ON THE BODY.

MAKES 250 ML

250 ml pink Himalayan salt crystals

3 drops ylang ylang essential oil

4 drops lavender essential oil

handful of dried pink roses, torn into small pieces

1. Place the sea salt and essential oils into a glass or plastic bowl and mix well to disperse the essential oils.
2. Add the dried rose petals and mix into the salt.
3. Spoon into sterilized plastic or glass containers.

How do I use the bath salts? Add a handful to the bath and disperse in the water. Agitate the water to dissolve the salt.

Groovy green and sunshine yellow bath salts

Magical bath fizzies

MAKES 4

250 ml bicarbonate of soda

50 ml citric acid

4 drops mandarin essential oil

4 drops lavender essential oil

20 ml mineral or filtered water

4 x soap moulds (or chocolate moulds)

4 x magic bean capsules (available
   from toy stores)

1. Place the bicarbonate of soda and citric acid in a plastic or glass bowl and mix together until most of the lumps have disappeared and the mixture resembles a fine powder.

2. Add the essential oils and mix well.

3. Add the water and mix together quickly until the mixture resembles damp sand. The mixture will fizz slightly – don't worry, this is normal!

4. Spoon some of the mixture into each of the moulds (about half full) and then place 1 magic bean capsule in the centre of each of the moulds.

5. Spoon some more mixture on top of the magic bean capsule, making sure that you cram as much mixture as you can into the mould – press firmly with the back of a metal tablespoon after each addition.

6. Allow to dry for 2 hours and then turn the mould upside down and gently tap to release the magical bath fizzy.

Funky fish bath soap

TURN BATH TIME INTO FUN TIME WITH CHARACTER SOAP BARS! YOU CAN USE ANY KIND OF HARD PLASTIC TOY TO PLACE
IN THE CENTRE OF THE CLEAR SOAP (I FOUND THESE PLASTIC FUNKY FISH SHAPES AT THE LOCAL PARTY SHOP).
I ALSO USED SOME DRIED WAKAME SEAWEED IN THE SOAP MOULDS TO GIVE THE SOAP A NATURAL SEA LOOK.
YOU CAN PURCHASE DRIED SEAWEED FROM ANY CHINESE SUPERMARKET.

MAKES 1 SOAP

90 g clear glycerine soap, cut into
   small blocks

20 drops lavender essential oil

pinch of dried wakame seaweed

1 x small square soap mould

1 x small plastic toy (in this case,
   a fish)

1. Place the blocks of glycerine soap in a saucepan over a very low heat until the soap has melted.

2. Add the essential oil and stir gently.

3. Place a pinch of dried seaweed into the soap mould (this makes the fish look like it is swimming amongst the seaweed in the ocean).

4. Pour half the mixture into the soap mould and allow to set slightly for about 10 minutes (just until the soap is firm).

5. Place the plastic toy on top of the 'set' soap in the centre of the mould. Pour the remaining melted soap over the toy.

6. Allow to set and become hard and only unmould the soap once it is cool. This should take about 1 hour.

Tip: If your child is getting impatient and can't wait to unmould the soap, place the soap in the fridge to speed up the process.

Funky fish bath soap

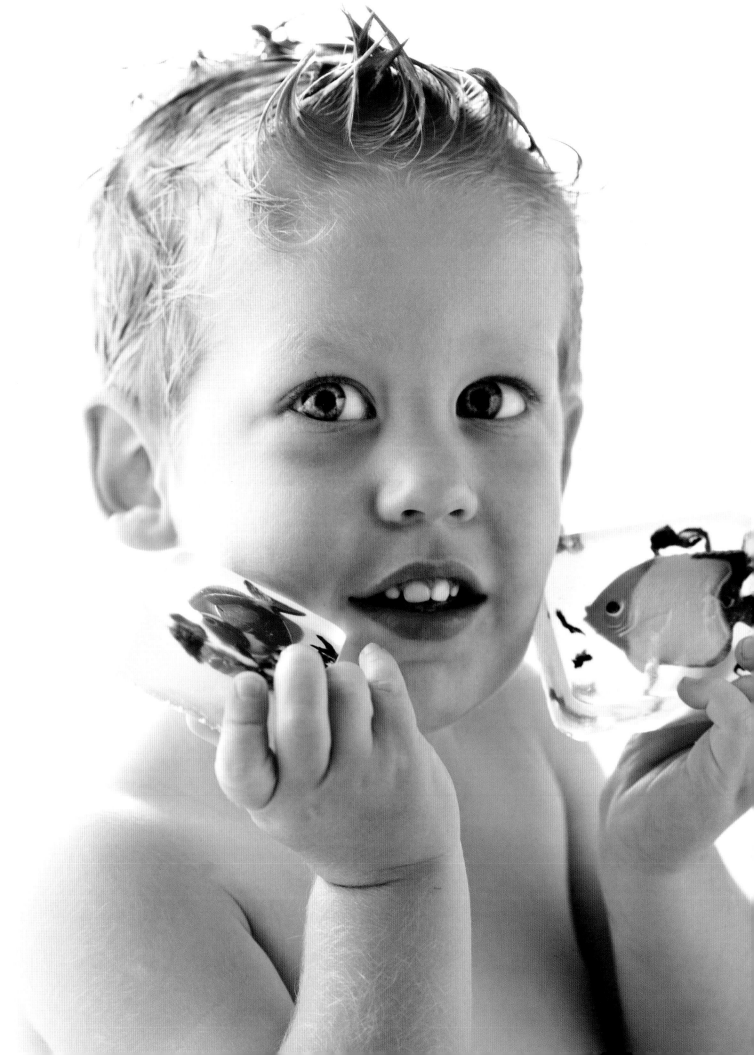

Soap

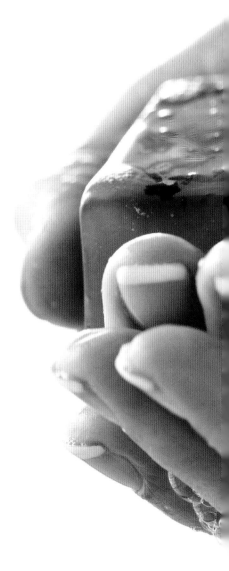

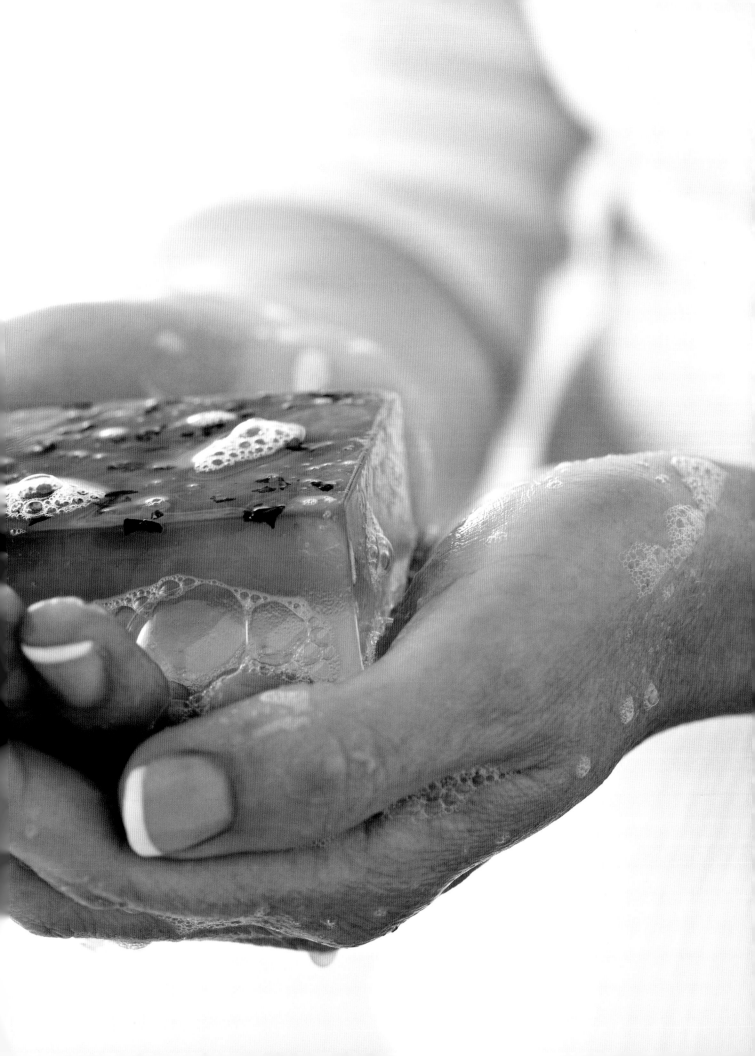

There are many different ways of making soap, and very different types of soap too! To make things easier and for the sake of brevity, I have included two of the most popular methods for making soap. Once you have tried these fantastic soap bars, you will never go back to using ordinary soap.

The first method is for a melt-and-pour type of soap, which is ready to use and the easiest method. The basic soap is unfragranced and all that you need to do is decide on the shape and which essential oils (or fragrance) to use. Herbal additives and tea are often added to give clear soap a natural golden colour, but other ingredients can be added to create texture and colour, for example oatmeal, poppy seeds or petals. This method is ideal for the novice soap-maker who wants to create instant soap that can be used immediately and is very easy to make.

The second method is for cold-processed soap, also known as true hand-made soap. This method is more suitable for the advanced soap-maker because the soap is created from scratch using oils, waxes and/or fat, as well as caustic soda. This method of soap making has to be extremely accurate and by using a digital scale it ensures flop-proof recipes. It is best to use a scale for both liquid and dry ingredients.

Care should be taken when using this method as it requires the addition of caustic chemicals. The caustic soda (also known as lye) is always added to the water and never the other way around. If water is added to the caustic soda, a small explosion could occur! But don't be afraid to try the recipes – just be very careful when adding the caustic soda.

Soap made using caustic soda is only ready for use after 6 weeks, when all traces of the caustic soda have naturally evaporated (along with the water). These soap bars are so gentle that they can be used on even the most sensitive skin.

I have included recipes for both cold-processed soap (which uses the cold-process method) as well as glycerine soap (melt-and-pour method).

Warning: Soap making is addictive … and fun … and creative!

SOAP MAKING SAFETY GUIDELINES:

Be very careful when mixing caustic soda into water. The caustic soda (sodium hydroxide) is very alkaline, and can cause serious chemical burns if it comes into contact with skin. If some mixture does spill onto the skin, immediately rinse with fresh water and then apply vinegar to neutralize the caustic soda.

Always wear protective eye wear, protective gloves and a protective face mask when using caustic soda.

Very important: add CAUSTIC SODA TO WATER and never the other way around!

Make sure that the area you are working in has adequate ventilation.

Store caustic soda in an area that is out of reach of children and pets.

Do not store caustic soda near food. It is also advisable to work in an area that is clear of foodstuffs when making soap.

When scraping and cleaning the saucepan (after soap making), place the leftover soap scrapings in a plastic bag and discard them. Wash the saucepan in hot, soapy water, always using gloves.

When handling and cutting soap that is still caustic remember to wear protective gloves, as the soap may cause a tingling sensation on the fingertips because not all the caustic soda has worked through the soap yet. The raw soap is still alkaline and will only be ready for use after 6 weeks.

SOME SOAPY TERMINOLOGY

Saponification: used to describe the chemical process that occurs when fats/oils and a caustic solution react together to form soap.

Trace: used to describe the stage of soap (usually when saponification occurs). The soap becomes thicker and more viscous, and has a 'thin custard' or 'sauce' consistency. You will notice that, when mixing the soap, if you lift the whisk or spoon the mixture will leave a visible trail.

Superfatting: when extra oil/butter is added to a soap recipe. By adding extra oil into your soap, you will end up with a much softer, gentler soap bar. It is advised to use no more than 10% total oil in the recipe (otherwise it may change the saponification value of the soap).

Saponification value: each oil has a certain saponification value (according to the density of each individual oil). The recipes have been formulated according to their saponification value so that the correct amount of sodium hydroxide (lye) is added within the recipe. Too much sodium hydroxide can be sensitizing on the skin, and too little sodium hydroxide can result in a 'fatty' or 'oily/greasy' feel to the soap.

Saponification chart: a standard chart is available online (www.fromnaturewithlove.com) to provide you with the saponification value of your specific oil. There are so many different oils to choose from, so if you do wish to replace any oils in cold-processed soap recipes you need to make sure that you have the correct saponification value and follow the instructions for converting your oil and changing your sodium hydroxide (lye) amount if necessary.

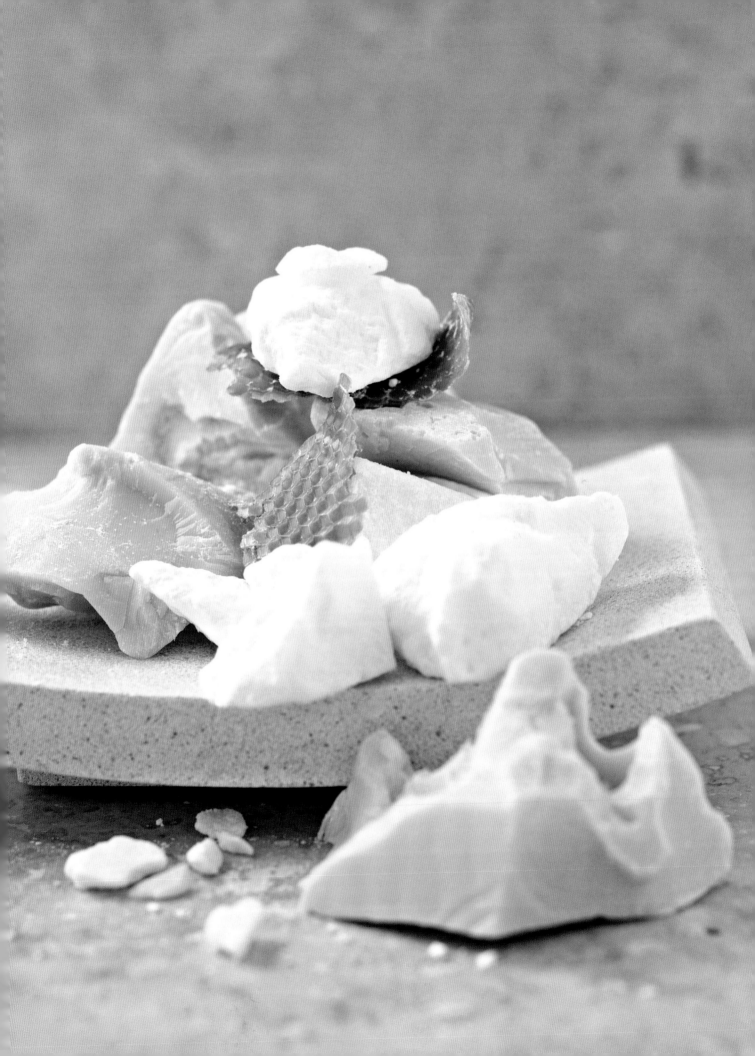

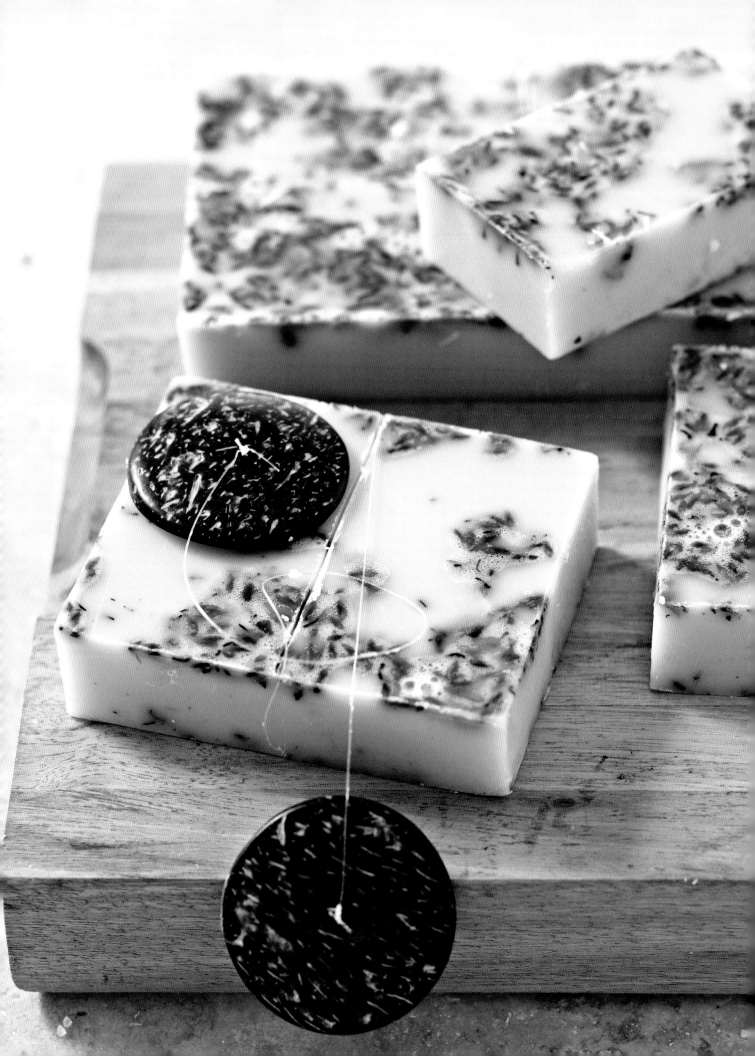

Basic soap-making techniques

SEE PAGE 20 FOR EQUIPMENT NEEDED TO MAKE GLYCERINE AND COLD-PROCESSED SOAP.
VISIT WWW.HOWTOMAKESOAP.CO.ZA FOR MORE INFORMATION ON HOW TO MAKE SOAP.

How to grease and unmould cold-processed soap

1. Grease your soap mould with some coconut oil or white margarine. Make sure that all the corners are greased well, so that the soap will turn out of the mould easily.
2. After making the soap mixture, pour into the greased mould and smooth the top.
3. Place the soap in the freezer for 1 hour.
4. Remove from the freezer and allow the soap to return to room temperature. Remove the protective plastic wrap from the soap.
5. Using rubber gloves (remember that the soap is still caustic), turn out the soap onto a plastic cutting board.

How to cut soap

(USING A SIMPLE TEMPLATE AND HOME-MADE SOAP-CUTTING TOOL)

1. You can also simply cut the soap with a non-serrated knife, but I find this method easier as it is less likely to cut skew soap bars.
2. First prepare a cutting template (you can re-use this template many times for cutting soap into equal-sized bars): use a piece of paper and cut to the size of the mould. Using a ruler, divide the template into 8 or 10 and mark into even-sized blocks.
3. Place the paper template over the soap, and lightly score the soap into bars according to the template markings.
4. Remove the template and turn the soap over. Repeat the process and score the markings onto the other side of the soap.
5. Use a piece of fishing gut (strong, clear nylon thread that you can also purchase from bead shops) and start by cutting the middle of the soap (creating two halves).
6. Wrap the clear thread around the markings and turn the soap over.
7. Pull in opposite directions, following the scored markings on the soap.

Glycerine soap

Green tea and lemongrass soap

LEMONGRASS HAS SUCH A STRONG CITRUS AROMA, WHICH IS PERFECT FOR SOAP.
THE GREEN TEA GIVES THE SOAP A NATURAL LIGHT GREEN-BROWN COLOUR.

MAKES 8 SOAP BARS

1 kg clear glycerine soap, roughly
  chopped into blocks
1 green tea bag (or 5 ml loose green
  tea leaves)
10 ml lemongrass essential oil

1. Melt the glycerine soap in a saucepan. Allow to melt slowly over low heat and do not stir the soap too often as this will lead to too much froth and bubbles in the mixture.
2. Add the green tea (if using a tea bag, cut open the tea bag and add the loose tea to the melted soap).
3. Allow the colour to develop slightly and stir gently.
4. Add the essential oil and mix gently.
5. Pour into a soap mould (I use a plastic square container that holds 1 kg of melted soap) and allow to cool completely.
6. Turn out and cut into 8 individual soap bars.
7. Wrap the soap bars in cellophane or tissue paper to preserve the fragrance.

Earl Grey and lemon soap

MAKES 8 SOAP BARS

1 kg clear glycerine soap, roughly
  chopped into blocks
1 Earl Grey tea bag (or 5 ml loose
  Earl Grey tea leaves)
10 ml bergamot essential oil
5 ml lemon essential oil

1. Melt the glycerine soap in a saucepan. Allow to melt slowly over low heat and do not stir the soap too often as this will lead to too much froth and bubbles in the mixture.
2. Add the Earl Grey tea (if using a tea bag, cut open the tea bag and add the loose tea leaves to the melted soap).
3. Allow the colour to develop slightly and stir gently.
4. Add the essential oils and mix gently.
5. Pour into a soap mould (I use a plastic square container that holds 1 kg of melted soap) and allow to cool completely.
6. Turn out and cut into 8 individual soap bars.
7. Wrap the soap bars in cellophane paper or tissue paper to preserve the fragrance.

Green tea and lemongrass soap

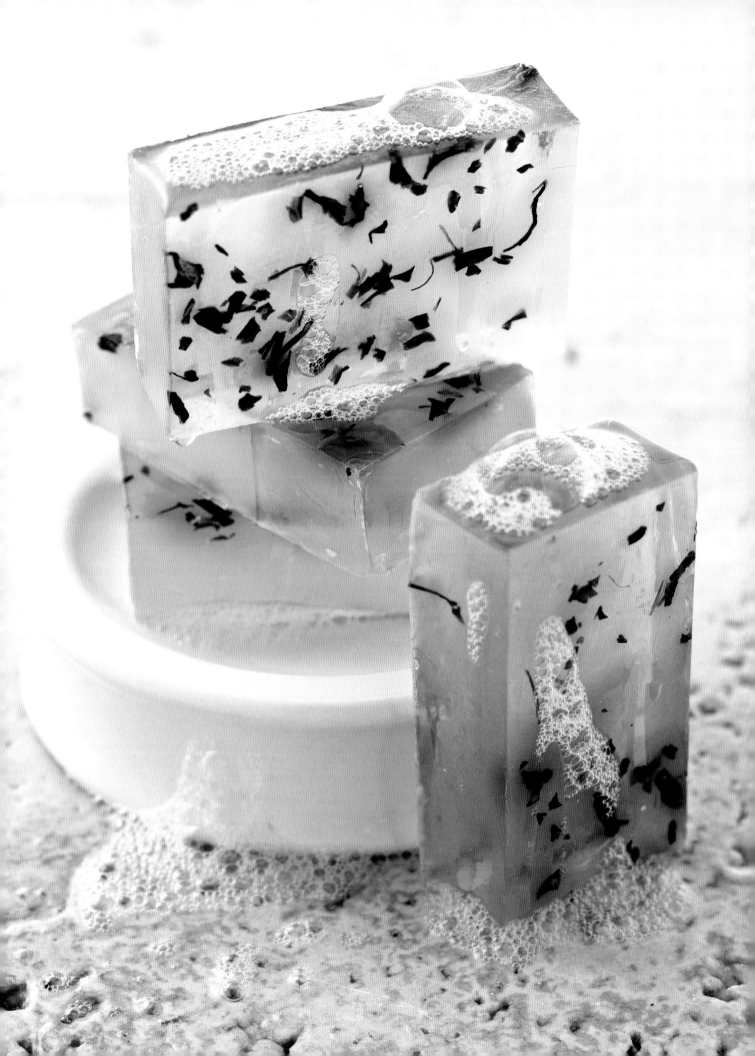

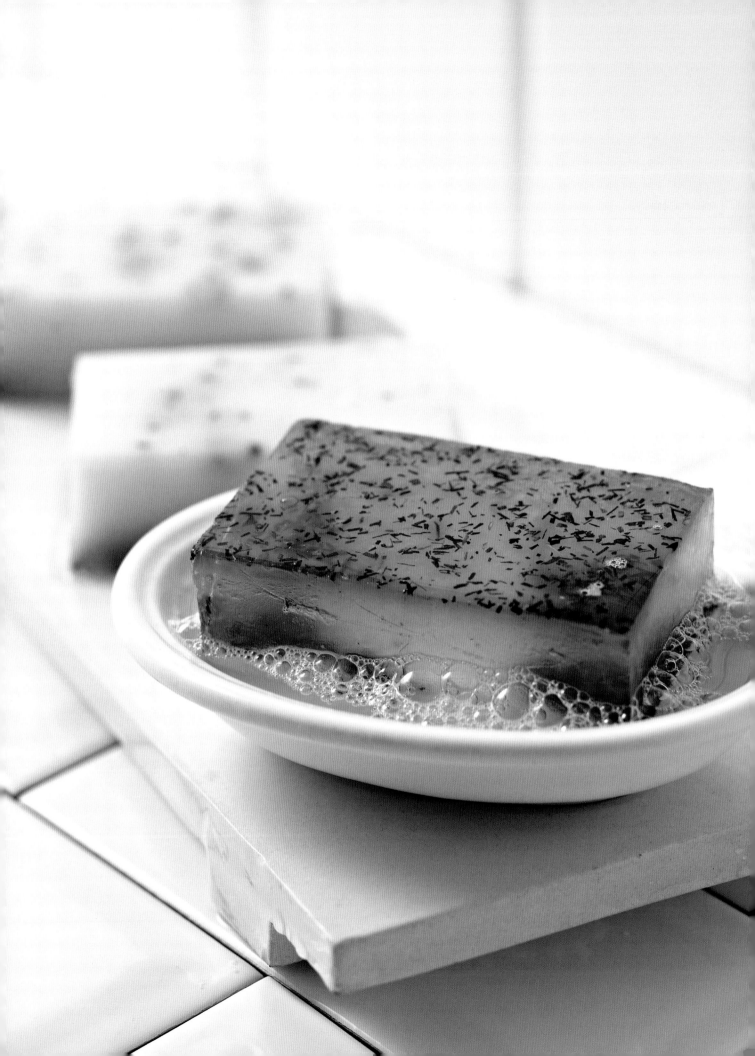

Rooibos and orange soap

MAKES 8 SOAP BARS

1 kg clear glycerine soap, roughly
    chopped into blocks

1 rooibos tea bag (or 5 ml loose rooibos
    tea leaves)

10 ml orange essential oil

5 ml lemongrass essential oil

1. Melt the glycerine soap in a saucepan. Allow to melt slowly over low heat and do not stir the soap too often as this will lead to too much froth and bubbles in the mixture.
2. Add the rooibos tea (if using a tea bag, cut open the tea bag and add the loose tea leaves to the melted soap).
3. Allow the colour to develop slightly and stir gently.
4. Add the essential oils and mix gently.
5. Pour into a soap mould (I use a plastic square container that holds 1 kg of melted soap) and allow to cool completely.
6. Turn out and cut into 8 individual soap bars.
7. Wrap the soap bars in cellophane paper or tissue paper to preserve the fragrance.

French lavender soap

MAKES 8 SOAP BARS

1 kg white glycerine soap, roughly
    chopped into blocks

15 ml dried lavender flowers

10 ml lavender essential oil

1. Melt the glycerine soap in a saucepan. Allow to melt slowly over low heat and do not stir the soap too often as this will lead to too much froth and bubbles in the mixture.
2. Add the dried lavender flowers and essential oil and stir gently.
3. Pour into a soap mould (I use a plastic square container that holds 1 kg of melted soap) and allow to cool completely.
4. Turn out and cut into 8 individual soap bars.
5. Wrap the soap bars in cellophane paper or tissue paper to preserve the fragrance.

Rooibos and orange soap

Rose geranium and poppy seed soap

MAKES 8 SOAP BARS

1 kg white glycerine soap, roughly
   chopped into blocks
5 ml cayenne pepper or a very tiny drop
   of red food colouring (for salmon pink
   colour – optional)
10 ml rose geranium essential oil
15 ml poppy seeds

1. Melt the glycerine soap in a saucepan. Allow to melt slowly over low heat and do not stir the soap too often as this will lead to too much froth and bubbles in the mixture.
2. Add the cayenne pepper or red food colouring (just a very small amount is needed – dip the tip of a cocktail stick into the colouring, and then add to the melted soap).
3. Allow the colour to develop slightly and stir gently.
4. Add the essential oil and poppy seeds and mix gently.
5. Pour into a soap mould (I use a plastic square container that holds 1 kg of melted soap) and allow to cool completely.
6. Turn out and cut into 8 individual soap bars.
7. Wrap the soap bars in cellophane paper or tissue paper to preserve the fragrance.

Orange flower, calendula and oat bran soap

MAKES 8 SOAP BARS

1 kg white glycerine soap, roughly
   chopped into blocks
30 ml oat bran
20 ml dried calendula petals
10 ml neroli essential oil
5 ml orange essential oil

1. Melt the glycerine soap in a saucepan. Allow to melt slowly over low heat and do not stir the soap too often as this will lead to too much froth and bubbles in the mixture.
2. Add the oat bran and calendula petals and stir gently.
3. Allow the colour to develop for about 2 minutes – the soap will turn a very pale beige colour.
4. Add the essential oils and mix gently.
5. Pour into a soap mould (I use a plastic square container that holds 1 kg of melted soap) and allow to cool completely.
6. Turn out and cut into 8 individual soap bars.
7. Wrap the soap bars in cellophane paper or tissue paper to preserve the fragrance.

Chamomile, honey and mandarin soap

MAKES 8 SOAP BARS

1kg white glycerine soap, roughly
   chopped into blocks
1 chamomile tea bag or 10 ml dried
   chamomile flowers
10 ml mandarin essential oil
5 ml Roman chamomile essential oil
5 ml honey

1. Melt the glycerine soap in a saucepan. Allow to melt slowly over low heat and do not stir the soap too often as this will lead to too much froth and bubbles in the mixture.
2. Add the chamomile tea (if using a tea bag, cut open the tea bag and add the loose tea leaves to the melted soap) or chamomile flowers.
3. Allow the colour to develop slightly and stir gently.
4. Add the essential oils and honey and mix gently.
5. Pour into a soap mould (I use a plastic square container that holds 1 kg of melted soap) and allow to cool completely.
6. Turn out and cut into 8 individual soap bars.
7. Wrap the soap bars in cellophane paper or tissue paper to preserve the fragrance.

From the top: Chamomile, honey and mandarine soap; Orange flower, calendula and oat bran soap; Rose geranium and poppy seed soap

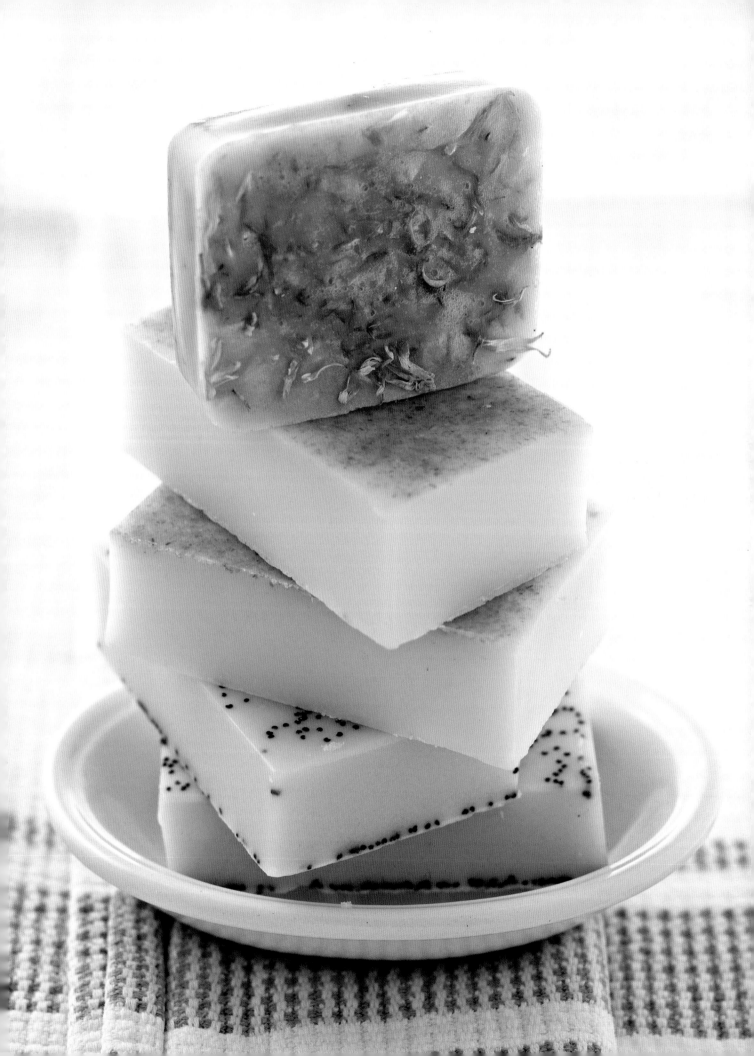

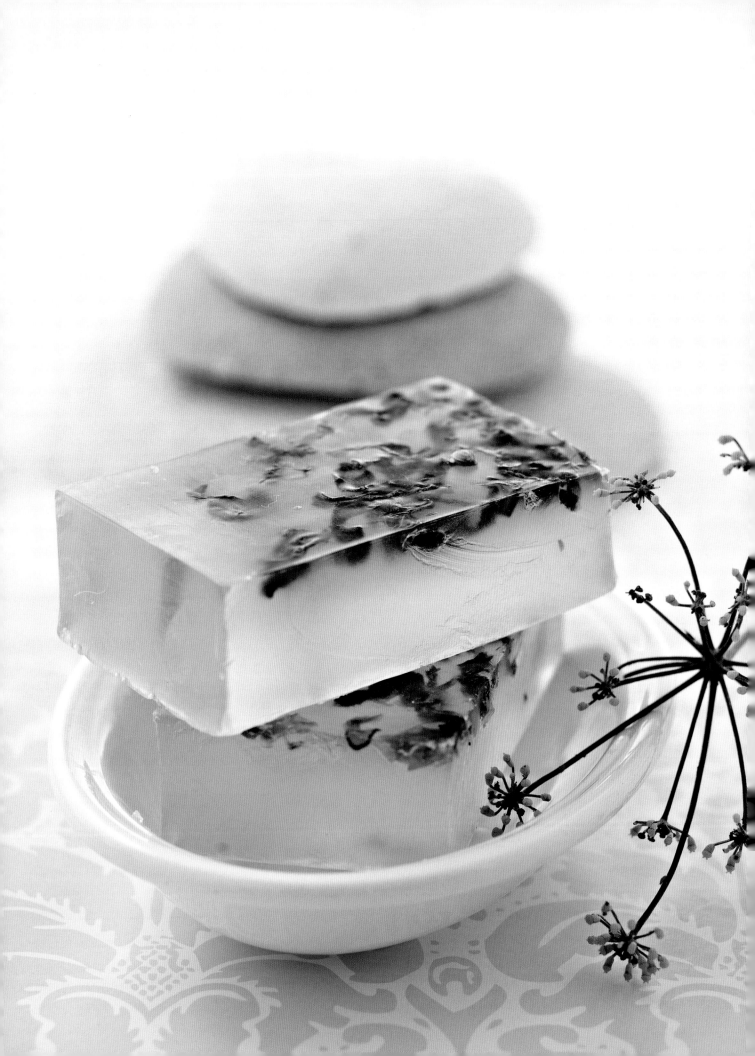

Basil and rosemary soap

MAKES 8 SOAP BARS

1 kg white glycerine soap, roughly
  chopped into blocks
10 ml dried basil or mixed herbs
10 ml basil essential oil
5 ml rosemary essential oil

1. Melt the glycerine soap in a saucepan. Allow to melt slowly over low heat and do not stir the soap too often as this will lead to too much froth and bubbles in the mixture.
2. Add the dried herbs and allow the colour to develop slightly.
3. Stir in the essential oils.
4. Pour into a soap mould (I use a plastic square container that holds 1 kg of melted soap) and allow to cool completely.
5. Turn out and cut into 8 individual soap bars.
6. Wrap the soap bars in cellophane paper or tissue paper to preserve the fragrance.

Fennel and seaweed soap

MAKES 8 SOAP BARS

1 kg clear glycerine soap, roughly
  chopped into blocks
10 ml dried seaweed
10 ml fennel essential oil
5 ml rosemary essential oil

1. Melt the glycerine soap in a saucepan. Allow to melt slowly over low heat and do not stir the soap too often as this will lead to too much froth and bubbles in the mixture.
2. Add the seaweed.
3. Add the essential oils and mix gently.
4. Pour into a soap mould (I use a plastic square container that holds 1 kg of melted soap) and allow to cool completely.
5. Turn out and cut into 8 individual soap bars.
6. Wrap the soap bars in cellophane paper or tissue paper to preserve the fragrance.

Peppermint and nettle soap

MAKES 8 SOAP BARS

1 kg white glycerine soap, roughly
  chopped into blocks
10 ml dried nettle or mixed herbs
10 ml peppermint essential oil

1. Melt the glycerine soap in a saucepan. Allow to melt slowly over low heat and do not stir the soap too often as this will lead to too much froth and bubbles in the mixture.
2. Add the dried nettles or herbs and stir gently. Allow the colour to develop slightly.
3. Add the essential oil and mix gently.
4. Pour into a soap mould (I use a plastic square container that holds 1 kg of melted soap) and allow to cool completely.
5. Turn out and cut into 8 individual soap bars.
6. Wrap the soap bars in cellophane paper or tissue paper to preserve the fragrance.

Fennel and seaweed soap

Cinnamon and cedarwood soap

MAKES 8 SOAP BARS

1 kg white glycerine soap, roughly
   chopped into blocks
15 ml ground cinnamon
10 ml cedarwood essential oil
5 ml cinnamon essential oil

1. Melt the glycerine soap in a saucepan. Allow to melt slowly over low heat and do not stir the soap too often as this will lead to too much froth and bubbles in the mixture.
2. Add the ground cinnamon. Allow the colour to develop slightly
3. Add the essential oils and mix gently.
4. Pour into a soap mould (I use a plastic square container that holds 1 kg of melted soap) and allow to cool completely.
5. Turn out and cut into 8 individual soap bars.
6. Wrap the soap bars in cellophane paper or tissue paper to preserve the fragrance.

Ginger, orange and coriander soap

MAKES 8 SOAP BARS

1 kg clear glycerine soap, roughly
   chopped into blocks
5 ml ground ginger
15 ml coriander seeds
10 ml orange essential oil
10 ml coriander essential oil
5 ml ginger essential oil

1. Melt the glycerine soap in a saucepan. Allow to melt slowly over low heat and do not stir the soap too often as this will lead to too much froth and bubbles in the mixture.
2. Add the ginger and the coriander seeds.
3. Add the essential oils and mix gently.
4. Pour into a soap mould (I use a plastic square container that holds 1 kg of melted soap) and allow to cool completely.
5. Turn out and cut into 8 individual soap bars.
6. Wrap the soap bars in cellophane paper or tissue paper to preserve the fragrance.

Coffee and sandalwood soap

MAKES 8 SOAP BARS

1 kg white glycerine soap, roughly
   chopped into blocks
30 ml dry ground coffee
10 ml cedarwood essential oil
5 ml sandalwood essential oil

1. Melt the glycerine soap in a saucepan. Allow to melt slowly over low heat and do not stir the soap too often as this will lead to too much froth and bubbles in the mixture.
2. Add the ground coffee and allow the colour to develop slightly, stirring very gently.
3. Add the essential oils and mix gently.
4. Pour into a soap mould (I use a plastic square container that holds 1 kg of melted soap) and allow to cool completely.
5. Turn out and cut into 8 individual soap bars.
6. Wrap the soap bars in cellophane paper or tissue paper to preserve the fragrance.

From left to right: *Ginger, orange and coriander soap;*
Cinnamon and cedarwood soap; Coffee and sandalwood soap

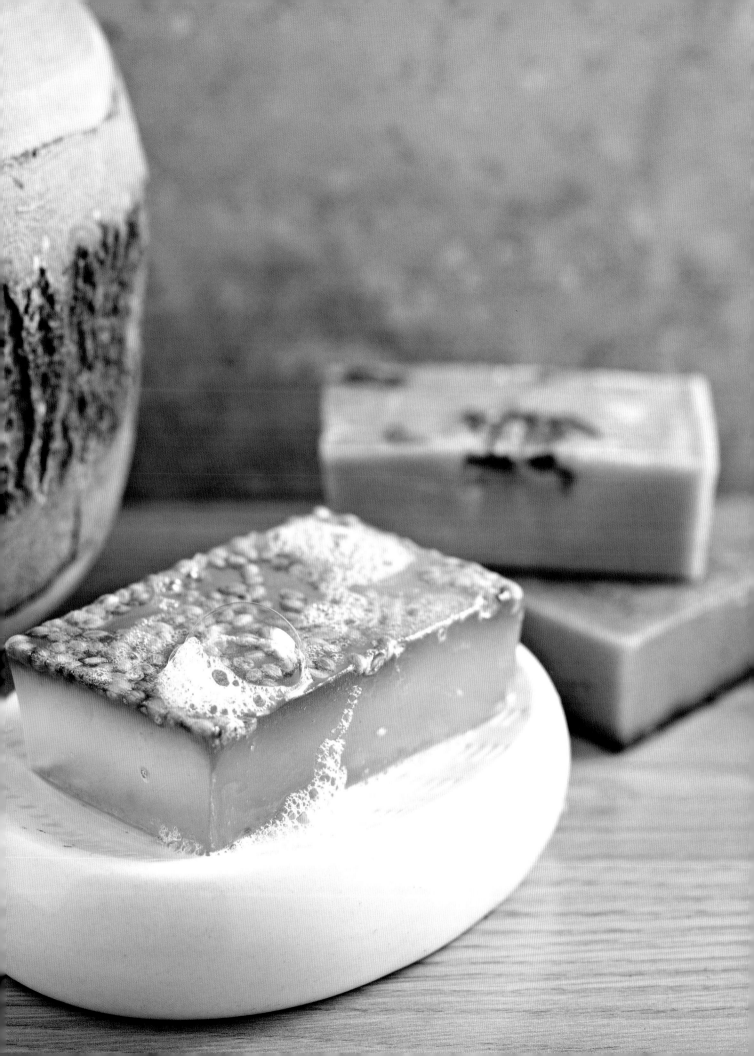

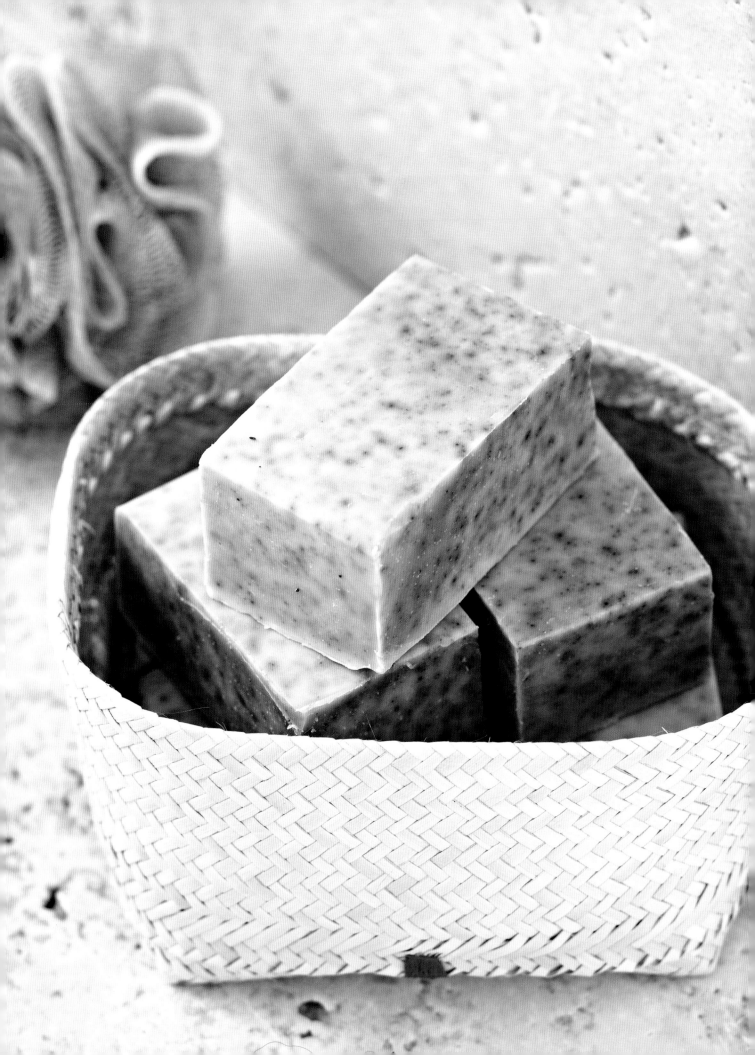

Cold-processed soap

Spirulina, basil and peppermint soap

MAKES 8 SOAP BARS

250 g white margarine
250 g coconut oil
250 g palm oil
250 g olive oil
340 g mineral or filtered water
144 g caustic soda (sodium hydroxide)
10 ml peppermint essential oil
10 ml eucalyptus essential oil
10 ml basil essential oil
50 ml spirulina powder
1 peppermint tea bag (optional)

1. Cut the white margarine, coconut oil and palm oil into small blocks. Add these blocks and the olive oil to an empty soap bucket or deep stainless-steel bowl.
2. Weigh off the correct amount of water (using a digital scale), and add to the second bucket or stainless-steel bowl.
3. Line the digital scale with some wax paper and weigh off the correct amount of caustic soda. Wearing protective eye goggles, gloves and a face mask, carefully add the caustic soda to the water.
4. Stir the caustic soda/water mixture with a long-handled spoon until the caustic soda is dissolved in the water – be careful, as this mixture gets very hot because of the chemical reaction.
5. Carefully add the caustic soda mixture to the bucket with the oils.
6. Mix with a whisk and then use a stick blender, using short bursts, until the mixture resembles thin custard and starts to trace.
7. Add the essential oils, spirulina powder and dried peppermint tea leaves to the soap mixture and mix again.
8. Pour the soap into the lined soap mould/or plastic container and cover with plastic wrap.
9. Cover with a piece of cardboard (or a stack of newspapers) and then cover with a blanket or an old towel.
10. Allow to set for 2 days and then remove from the soap mould. Remember to wear gloves when handling the soap as it is still caustic.
11. Place the soap on a plastic cutting board and cut into blocks. Allow the soap to cure for 6 weeks. Turn the soap every week or so and keep covered until ready to use.
12. After 6 weeks the soap will have no traces of caustic soda and will be the correct pH for your skin.

CAUTION: Do not use the soap for at least 6 weeks as it will still contain traces of caustic soda.

Spirulina, basil and peppermint soap

Lemongrass and rosemary olive oil soap

MAKES 8 SOAP BARS

830 g olive oil

20 g sunflower oil

58 g beeswax

285 g mineral or filtered water

112 g caustic soda (sodium hydroxide)

10 ml lemongrass essential oil

10 ml rosemary essential oil

2 tablespoons dried rosemary leaves,
   finely chopped

1. Heat the olive oil, sunflower oil and beeswax together in a saucepan over very gentle heat until the beeswax has melted. Pour into an empty soap bucket or deep stainless-steel bowl.

2. Weigh off the correct amount of water and pour into the second plastic soap bucket or stainless-steel bowl.

3. Line the digital scale with some wax paper and weigh off the correct amount of caustic soda. Wearing protective eye goggles, gloves and a face mask, carefully add the caustic soda to the water.

4. Stir the caustic soda/water mixture with a long-handled spoon until the caustic soda is dissolved in the water – be careful, as this mixture gets very hot because of the chemical reaction.

5. Place a sugar thermometer in the bucket or glass jug containing the caustic soda and water.

6. Place another sugar thermometer in the saucepan containing the melted oils and beeswax.

7. When both thermometers have reached about the same temperature (ideally between 50 and 60 °C), add the caustic soda solution to the melted oils.

8. Mix with a whisk and then use a stick blender, using short bursts, until the mixture resembles thin custard and starts to trace.

9. Add the essential oils and the rosemary leaves to the soap mixture and mix again.

10. Pour the soap into the lined soap mould/or plastic container and cover with plastic wrap.

11. Cover with a piece of cardboard (or a stack of newspapers) and then cover with a blanket or an old towel.

12. Allow to set for 2 days and then remove from the soap mould. Remember to wear gloves when handling the soap as it is still caustic.

13. Place the soap on a plastic cutting board and cut into blocks. Allow the soap to cure for 6 weeks. Turn the soap every week or so and keep covered until ready to use.

14. After 6 weeks the soap will have no traces of caustic soda and will be the correct pH for your skin.

CAUTION: Do not use the soap for at least 6 weeks as it will still contain traces of caustic soda.

Lemongrass and rosemary olive oil soap
Top left to right: *Adding caustic soda to mineral or filtered water;*
Checking temperature of caustic soda solution and melted oils using a thermometer
Bottom left to right: *Adding caustic soda to melted oils when they have reached the same temperature;*
Mixing in essential oils and dried rosemary when mixture has reached trace stage.

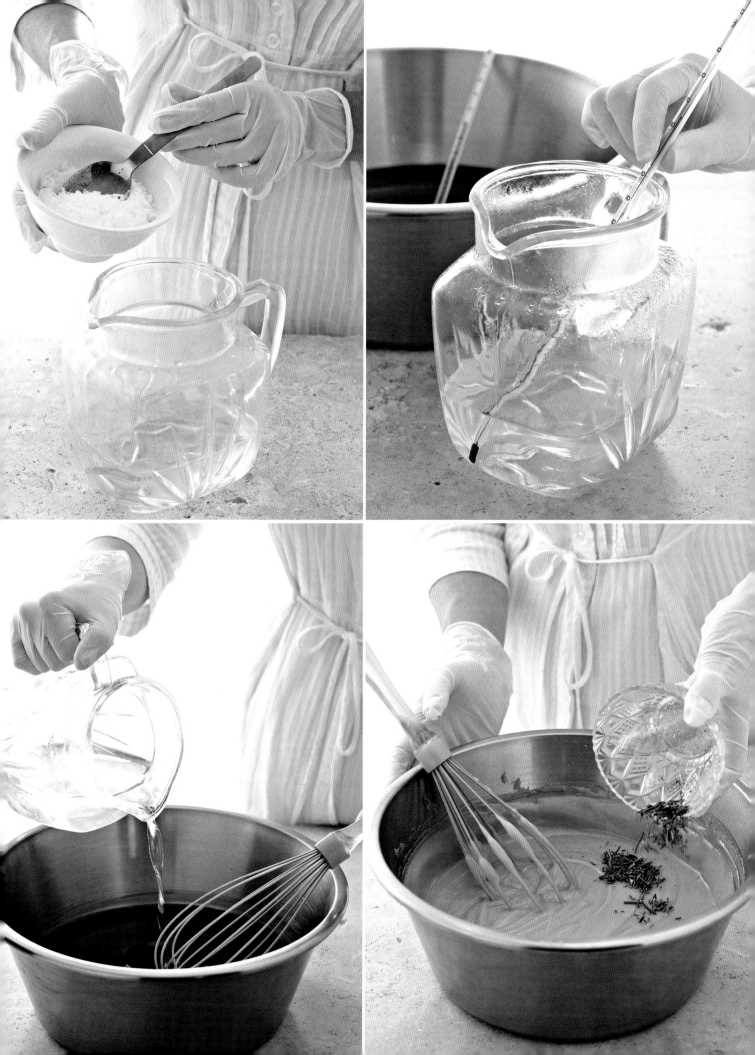

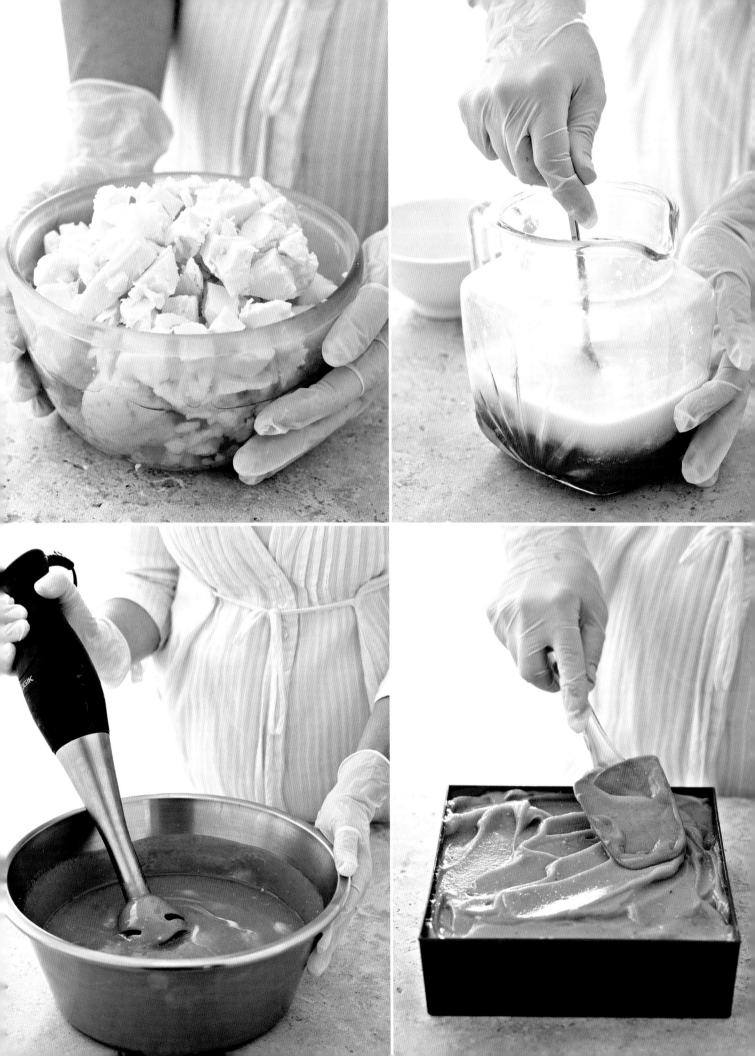

Creamy vanilla and goat's milk soap

THIS IS A LUXURIOUS, CREAMY SOAP BAR. IF FRESH GOAT'S MILK IS UNAVAILABLE, USE POWDERED GOAT'S MILK MIXED WITH MINERAL OR FILTERED WATER. I MANAGED TO FIND A GOOD-QUALITY POWDERED GOAT'S MILK FROM MY LOCAL HEALTH SHOP.

MAKES 8 SOAP BARS

250 g white margarine
20 g shea butter
250 g palm oil
250 g coconut oil
250 g sunflower oil
330 g goat's milk
144 g caustic soda (sodium hydroxide)
1 vanilla pod
10 ml ylang ylang essential oil
10 ml neroli essential oil

1. Cut the white margarine, shea butter and palm oil into small blocks. Add these blocks and the coconut and sunflower oils to an empty soap bucket or deep stainless-steel bowl.
2. Weigh off the correct amount of goat's milk (or goat's milk powder and water solution), and place into the second soap bucket or stainless-steel bowl.
3. Line the digital scale with some wax paper and weigh off the correct amount of caustic soda. Wearing protective eye goggles, gloves and a face mask, carefully add the caustic soda to the goat's milk.
4. Stir the caustic soda/goat's milk mixture with a long-handled spoon until the caustic soda is dissolved in the water – be careful, as this mixture gets very hot because of the chemical reaction.
5. Carefully add the caustic soda/goat's milk mixture to the bucket with the oils.
6. Mix with a whisk and then use a stick blender, using short bursts, until the mixture resembles thin custard and starts to trace.
7. You will notice that the mixture has turned a lovely caramel, buttery vanilla colour – don't panic because this is normal, and is only due to the addition of the milk.
8. Split the vanilla pod in half lengthways, and scrape out all that gooey vanilla paste.
9. Add the essential oils and the vanilla paste to the soap mixture and mix again.
10. Pour the soap into the lined soap mould/or plastic container and cover with plastic wrap.
11. Cover with a piece of cardboard (or a stack of newspapers) and then cover with a blanket or an old towel.
12. Allow to set for 2 days and then remove from the soap mould. Remember to wear gloves when handling the soap as it is still caustic.
13. Place the soap on a plastic cutting board and cut into blocks. Allow the soap to cure for 6 weeks. Turn the soap every week or so and keep covered until ready to use.
14. After 6 weeks the soap will have no traces of caustic soda and will be the correct pH for your skin.

CAUTION: Do not use the soap for at least 6 weeks as it will still contain traces of caustic soda.

Creamy vanilla and goat's milk soap
Top left to right: White margarine, shea butter, palm oil, coconut and sunflower oil;
Stirring the caustic soda/goat's milk mixture with a long-handled spoon until caustic soda has dissolved
Bottom left to right: Mixing with a stick blender until the mixture begins to thicken;
Pouring soap into lined soap mould, using a spatula to smooth the top

Rooibos and lemongrass delight

MAKES 8 SOAP BARS

330 g mineral or filtered water

2 rooibos tea bags

30 ml honey

250 g white margarine

250 g coconut oil

250 g palm oil

250 g sunflower oil

144 g caustic soda (sodium hydroxide)

20 ml lemongrass essential oil

1. Boil the water and add the rooibos tea bags. Allow to cool and then remove the tea bags. (Keep 1 used teabag so that you can add the loose tea leaves to the soap later). Stir in the honey.
2. Cut the white margarine, coconut oil and palm oil into small blocks. Add these blocks and the sunflower oil to an empty soap bucket or deep stainless-steel bowl.
3. Weigh off 330 g of the cooled rooibos tea, and add to the second bucket or stainless-steel bowl.
4. Line the digital scale with some wax paper and weigh off the correct amount of caustic soda. Wearing protective eye goggles, gloves and a face mask, carefully add the caustic soda to the cooled rooibos tea.
5. Stir the caustic soda/tea mixture with a long-handled spoon until the caustic soda is dissolved in the cooled tea mixture – be careful, as this mixture gets very hot because of the chemical reaction.
6. Add the caustic soda/tea mixture to the bucket with the oils.
7. Mix with a whisk and then use a stick blender, using short bursts, until the mixture resembles thin custard and starts to trace.
8. Add the essential oil and the loose rooibos tea leaves to the soap mixture and mix again.
9. Pour the soap into the lined soap mould/or plastic container and cover with plastic wrap.
10. Cover with a piece of cardboard (or a stack of newspapers) and then cover with a blanket or an old towel.
11. Allow to set for 2 days and then remove from the soap mould. Remember to wear gloves when handling the soap as it is still caustic.
12. Place the soap on a plastic cutting board and cut into blocks. Allow the soap to cure for 6 weeks. Turn the soap every week or so and keep covered until ready to use.
13. After 6 weeks the soap will have no traces of caustic soda and will be the correct pH for your skin.

CAUTION: Do not use the soap for at least 6 weeks as it will still contain traces of caustic soda.

Rooibos and lemongrass delight

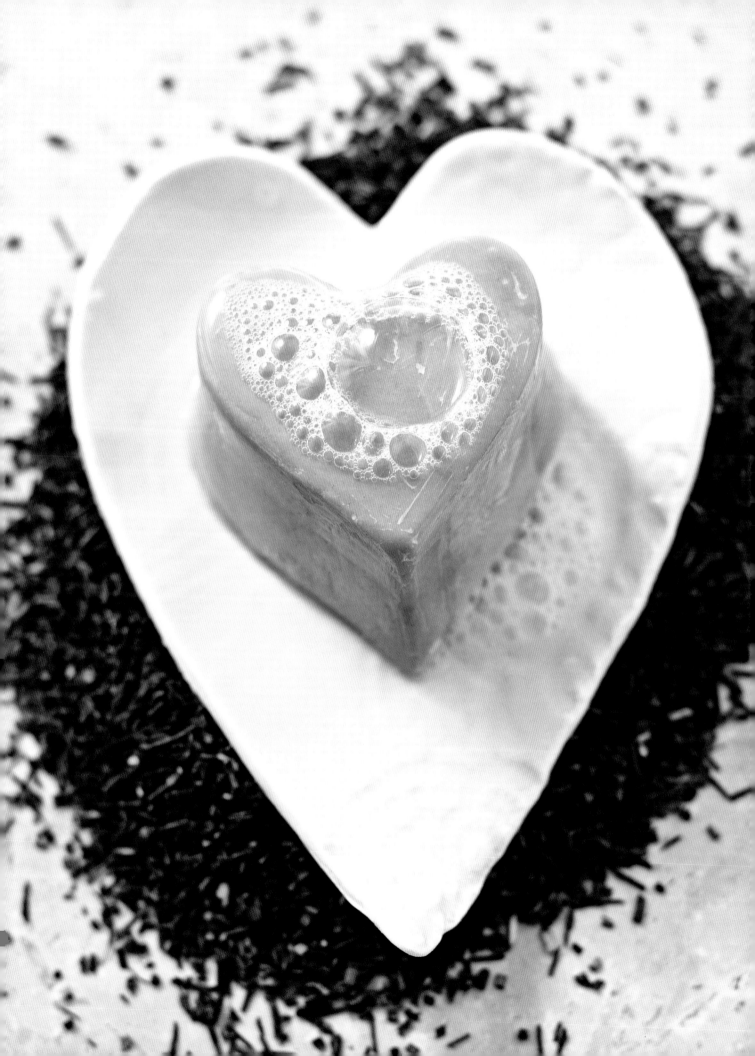

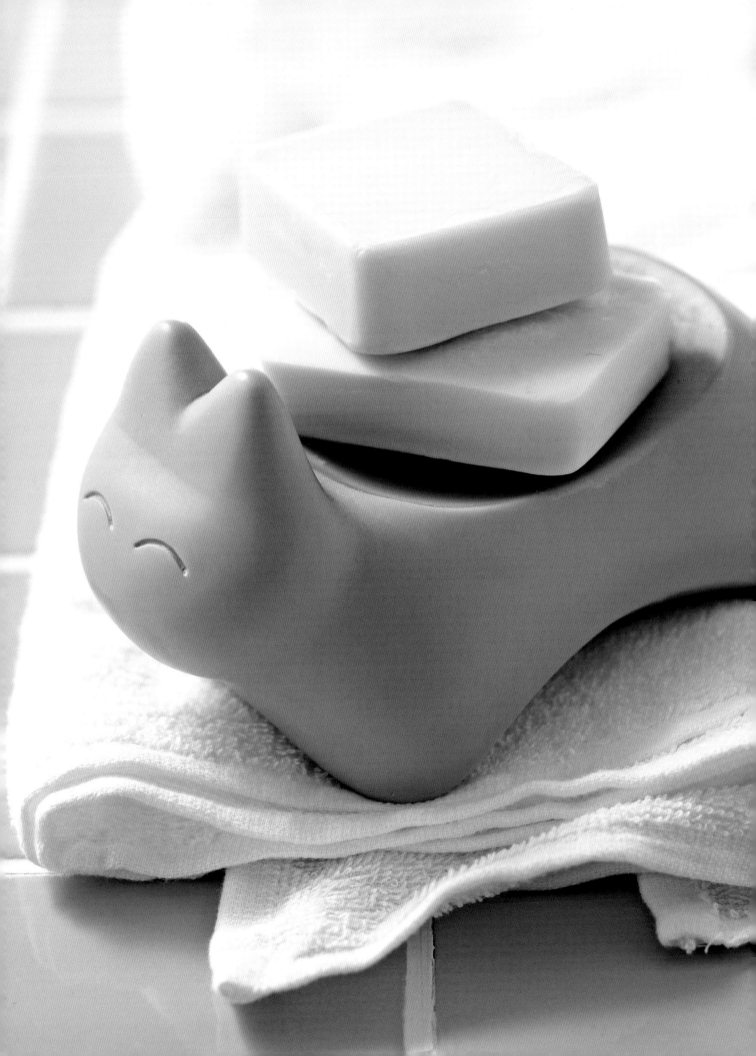

Baby soap bar with lavender, rose geranium and calendula

MAKES 8 SOAP BARS

250 g white margarine

250 g coconut oil

250 g sunflower oil

250 g grapeseed oil

58 g beeswax

330 g mineral or filtered water

149 g caustic soda (sodium hydroxide)

10 ml calendula essential oil (or 10 ml calendula-infused oil, see page 146)

10 ml organic rose geranium essential oil

10 ml organic lavender essential oil

1. Weigh the margarine, oils and beeswax and place into a large saucepan. Heat gently until the beeswax has melted completely.
2. As soon as the beeswax has melted, remove the saucepan from the heat and pour the mixture into an empty plastic bucket or deep stainless-steel bowl.
3. Weigh off the correct amount of water and pour into the second plastic soap bucket or stainless-steel bowl.
4. Line the digital scale with some wax paper and weigh off the correct amount of caustic soda. Wearing protective eye goggles, gloves and a face mask, carefully add the caustic soda to the water.
5. Stir the caustic soda/water mixture with a long-handled spoon until the caustic soda is dissolved in the water – be careful, as this mixture gets very hot because of the chemical reaction.
6. Place a sugar thermometer in the bucket containing the caustic soda and water.
7. Place another sugar thermometer in the saucepan containing the melted oils and beeswax.
8. When both thermometers have reached about the same temperature (ideally between 50 and 60 °C), add the caustic soda solution to the melted oils.
9. Mix with a whisk and then use a stick blender, using short bursts, until the mixture resembles thin custard and starts to trace.
10. Add the essential oils to the soap mixture and mix again.
11. Pour the soap into the lined soap mould/or plastic container and cover with plastic wrap.
12. Cover with a piece of cardboard (or a stack of newspapers) and then cover with a blanket or an old towel.
13. Allow to set for 2 days and then remove from the soap mould. Remember to wear gloves when handling the soap as it is still caustic.
14. Place the soap on a plastic cutting board and cut into blocks. Allow the soap to cure for 6 weeks. Turn the soap every week or so and keep covered until ready to use.
15. After 6 weeks the soap will have no traces of caustic soda and will be the correct pH for your skin.

CAUTION: Do not use the soap for at least 6 weeks as it will still contain traces of caustic soda.

Baby soap bar with lavender, rose geranium and calendula

Men's shaving soap bar with cedarwood, sandalwood and lavender

MY MALE CLIENTS ABSOLUTELY RAVE ABOUT THIS CREAMY, LOW-FOAMING SOAP BAR. THE SOAP GIVES A TREMENDOUS AMOUNT OF SLIP FOR SHAVING, WITHOUT THE HARSH CHEMICAL INGREDIENTS SUCH AS ARTIFICIAL FRAGRANCE AND PROPELLANTS USED IN COMMERCIAL SHAVING CREAMS AND GELS. PERFECT FOR SENSITIVE SKIN. THE LAVENDER, SANDALWOOD AND CEDARWOOD ESSENTIAL OILS SOOTHE IRRITATION CAUSED BY SHAVING.

MAKES 8 SOAP BARS

850 g olive oil

10 g shea butter

58 g beeswax

285 g mineral or filtered water

112 g caustic soda (sodium hydroxide)

10 ml cedarwood essential oil

10 ml sandalwood essential oil

10 ml lavender essential oil

1. Heat the olive oil, shea butter and beeswax together in a saucepan. Heat very gently until the beeswax has melted.
2. As soon as the beeswax has melted, remove the saucepan from the heat and pour the mixture into an empty plastic bucket or deep stainless-steel bowl.
3. Weigh off the correct amount of water and pour into a large, clean plastic soap bucket or stainless-steel bowl.
4. Line the digital scale with some wax paper and weigh off the correct amount of caustic soda. Wearing protective eye goggles, gloves and a face mask, carefully add the caustic soda to the water.
5. Stir the caustic soda/water mixture with a long-handled spoon until the caustic soda is dissolved in the water – be careful, as this mixture gets very hot because of the chemical reaction.
6. Place a sugar thermometer in the bucket or glass jug containing the caustic soda and water.
7. Place another sugar thermometer in the saucepan containing the melted oils and beeswax.
8. When both thermometers have reached about the same temperature (ideally between 50 and 60 °C), add the caustic soda/water solution to the melted oils.
9. Mix with a whisk and then use a stick blender, using short bursts, until the mixture resembles thin custard and starts to trace.
10. Add the essential oils to the soap mixture and mix again.
11. Pour the soap into the lined soap mould/or plastic container and cover with plastic wrap.
12. Cover with a piece of cardboard (or a stack of newspapers) and then cover with a blanket or an old towel.
13. Allow to set for 2 days and then remove from the soap mould. Remember to wear gloves when handling the soap as it is still caustic.
14. Place the soap on a plastic cutting board and cut into blocks. Allow the soap to cure for 6 weeks. Turn the soap every week or so and keep covered until ready to use.
15. After 6 weeks the soap will have no traces of caustic soda and will be the correct pH for your skin.

CAUTION: Do not use the soap for at least 6 weeks as it will still contain traces of caustic soda.

Men's shaving soap bar with cedarwood, sandalwood and lavender

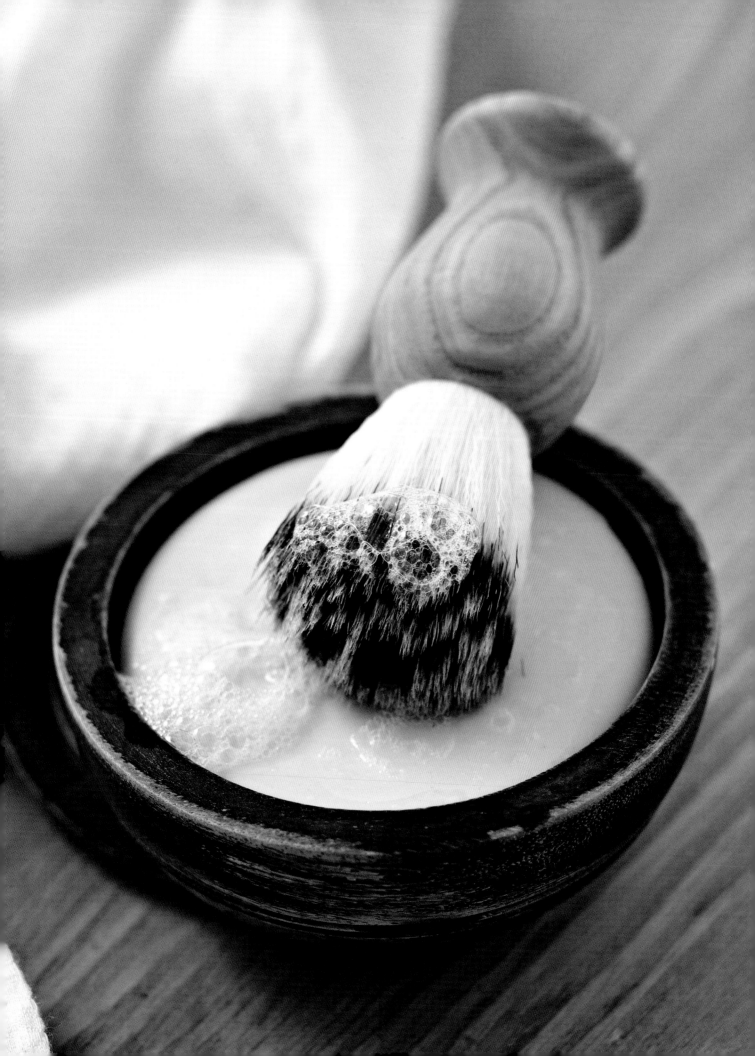

Products for your home

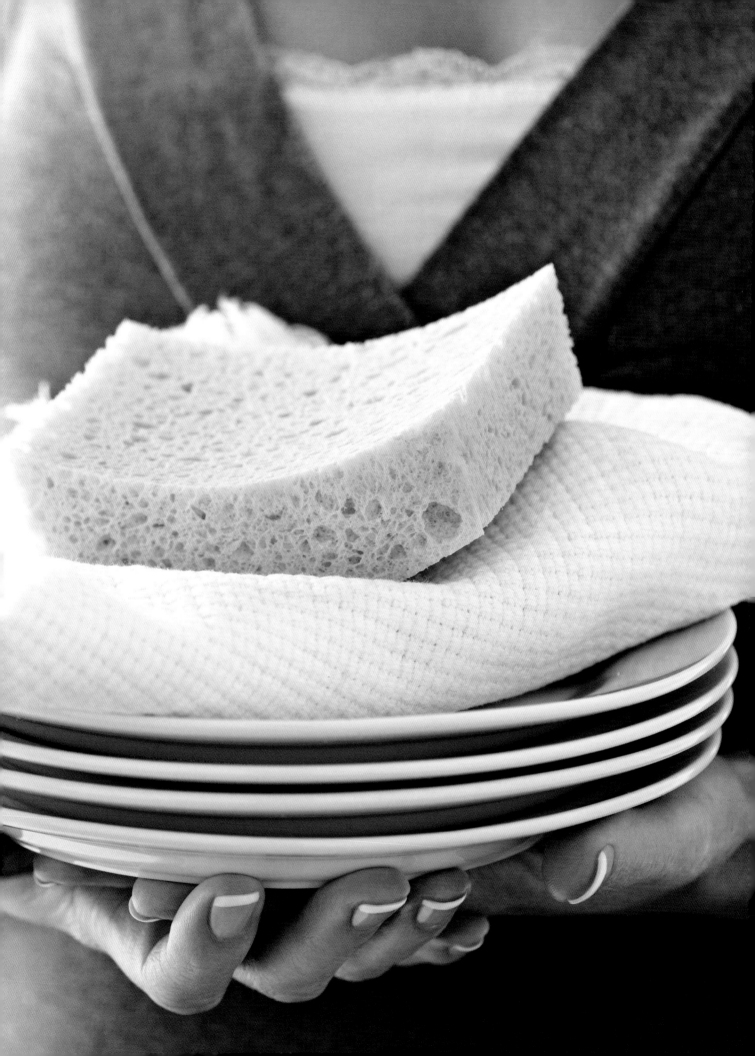

All-purpose cleanser

USE THIS NATURAL ALL-PURPOSE CLEANSER TO CLEAN BATHROOMS AND BASINS. IT CONTAINS NO AMMONIA OR HARSH CHEMICALS, AND HAS ANTI-BACTERIAL PROPERTIES TOO! THE KAOLIN CLAY HELPS TO BIND DIRT AND GRIME AND THE SURFACTANT/SOAP BASE HELPS TO STRIP AWAY GREASE. THIS NATURAL CLEANSER REQUIRES A BIT OF ELBOW GREASE BECAUSE THERE ARE NO HARSH CHEMICALS TO DISSOLVE AWAY THE DIRT. RINSE WELL TO REMOVE ALL RESIDUE AFTER USE.

MAKES 1 LITRE

500 ml kaolin clay
900 ml filtered water
100 ml concentrated unsweetened
   lemon juice or freshly squeezed
   lemon juice (strain to remove pips)
50 ml surfactant base (unfragranced
   liquid soap base)
2.5 ml xanthan gum (optional)
40 drops citronella essential oil
25 drops pine essential oil

1. Mix all the ingredients together and blend well with a whisk. Leave for 5 minutes and then whisk again well. Leave for another 10 minutes and whisk once more.
2. Pour into an empty household cleanser container with a re-sealable lid.

How do I use the cleanser? Apply to a wet cloth or sponge and wipe the bathtub or basin. Rinse well with clean water.

Tip: The xanthan gum is available from health shops and pharmacies. It is relatively inexpensive, and it helps to thicken the mixture. If you don't have xanthan gum, simply omit it. Your mixture will be as effective, only thinner.

Multi-purpose kitchen and surface cleanser

THIS RECIPE IS SIMILAR TO DISHWASHING LIQUID, BUT IT IS MORE DILUTED SO THAT THE LIQUID IS LESS SOAPY. IT CAN BE USED TO WIPE KITCHEN COUNTERS, CLEAN BATHROOMS AND SHOWERS AS WELL FLOORS.

MAKES 500 ML

250 ml surfactant base (unfragranced
   liquid soap base)
250 ml filtered water
20 drops lavender essential oil
10 drops lemon essential oil
20 drops tea tree essential oil

1. Mix all the ingredients together and stir with a metal spoon until combined. Pour into an empty household cleanser container with a re-sealable lid.

How do I use the cleanser? Use on all surfaces to clean and to wipe down kitchen counters. To clean floors, dilute 5 ml cleanser in 5 litres of warm water. Do not use too much cleanser because it will make the floors sticky.

All-purpose cleanser and
Multi-purpose kitchen and surface cleanser

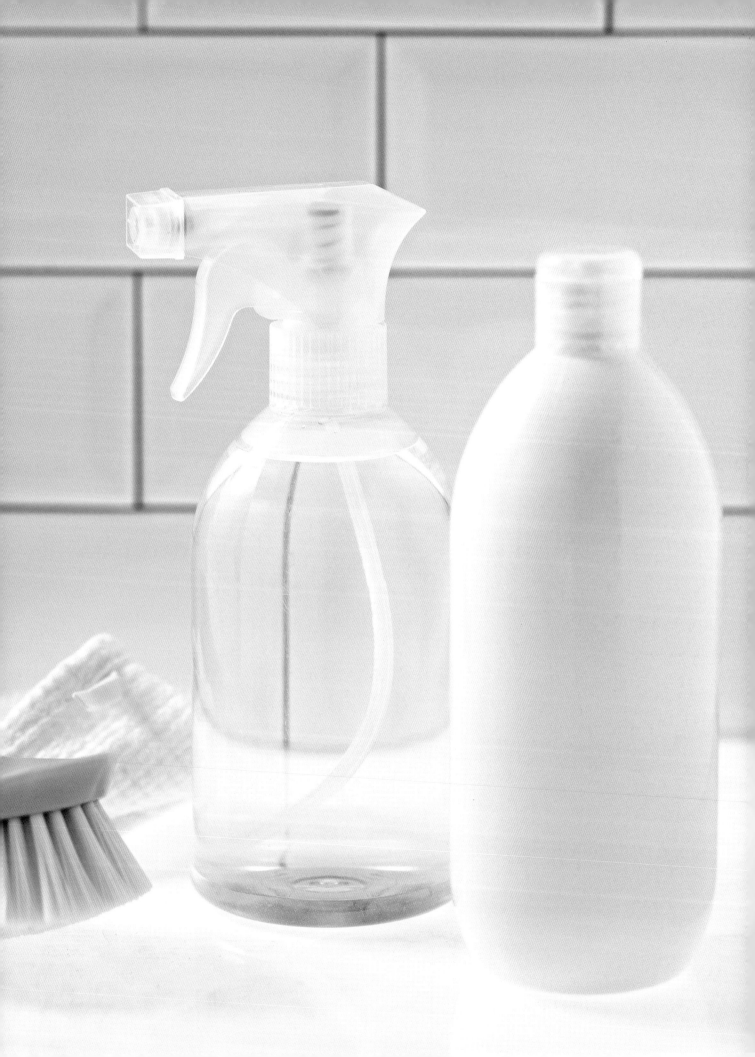

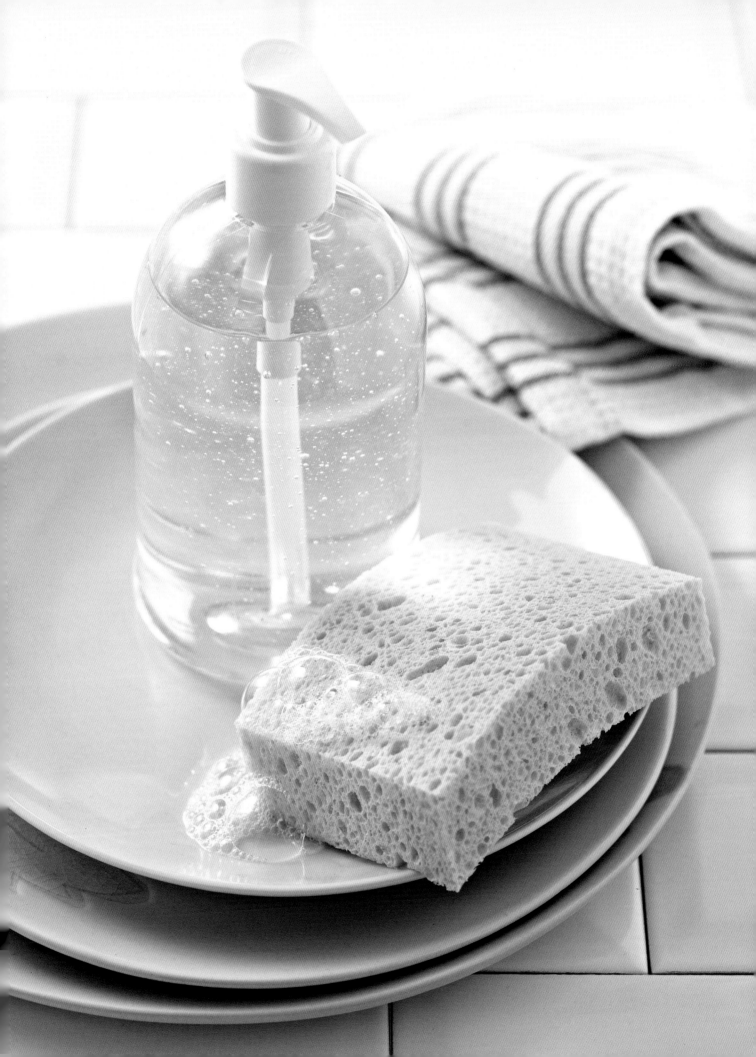

Grapefruit and lime dishwashing liquid

THIS FOAMING WASHING LIQUID IS GENTLER ON THE HANDS THAN CONVENTIONAL DISHWASHING LIQUID. I LIKE TO USE ZINGY CITRUS, WHICH HELPS TO CLEAN THE DISHES AND LEAVES A WONDERFUL LEMON SCENT IN THE KITCHEN.

MAKES 500 ML

350 ml surfactant base (unfragranced
    liquid soap base)
150 ml filtered water
20 drops grapefruit essential oil
20 drops lime essential oil
10 drops lemongrass essential oil

1. Mix all the ingredients together and stir with a metal spoon until combined. Pour into an empty household cleanser container with a re-sealable lid.

How do I use the dishwashing liquid? Add a little to a sinkful of warm water to wash glasses, cutlery and crockery.

Aromatherapy washing liquid

THIS IS A FOAMING LIQUID THAT CAN BE USED FOR WASHING YOUR CLOTHES. ROSEMARY, LEMONGRASS AND LAVENDER GIVE THE WATER A GENTLE AND REFRESHING NATURAL AROMA. A LITTLE GOES A LONG WAY, SO BE CAREFUL NOT TO USE TOO MUCH IN YOUR WASHING MACHINE.

MAKES 1 LITRE

1 litre surfactant base (unfragranced
    liquid soap base)
50 ml filtered water
30 drops lavender essential oil
20 drops rosemary essential oil
15 drops lemongrass essential oil

1. Mix all the ingredients together and stir with a metal spoon until combined. Pour into a storage bottle.

How do I use the washing liquid? Use about 30 ml washing liquid for a single load of washing.

Did you know? Surfactants are the name used to describe the active ingredient in most detergents (including other soap-like products such as foam bath, body wash and shampoo). The molecular structure of surfactants allows it to be soluble in water, oil or fat. This means that when surfactants are added to water they help to lower the surface tension and are capable of emulsifying oils into the water. Surfactants are also called wetting agents, and are said to make water 'wetter'. This is why grease and grime are easier to remove from fabric when washing clothes with a detergent and when washing your skin with soap.

Grapefruit and lime dishwashing liquid

Classic linen spray

MAKES 200 ML

200 ml filtered water
20 drops lavender essential oil

1. Pour the water and essential oil into a 200 ml spray bottle and shake well.
2. Shake the mixture daily and, after 1 week, decant the mixture and strain it through a muslin cloth.
3. Re-bottle the mixture and shake well before use.

How do I use the linen spray? Spray directly onto fabrics for a wonderful lavender aroma.
Caution: Spray at least 15 cm away from the fabric. Do not use citrus oils as they have a yellow or orange colour that can stain fabric.

Spring clean aromatherapy air-freshener

MAKES 200 ML

200 ml filtered water
15 drops lavender essential oil
15 drops cedarwood essential oil
20 drops rose geranium essential oil
10 drops ylang ylang essential oil
5 drops lemongrass essential oil

1. Pour the water and essential oils into a 200 ml spray bottle and shake well.
2. Shake the mixture daily and, after 1 week, decant the mixture and strain it through a muslin cloth.
3. Re-bottle the mixture and shake well before use.

How do I use the air-freshener? Shake well before use. Spray into the room to refresh the air and to release a spring-clean aroma throughout your home.

Citrus fresh room spray

MAKES 200 ML

200 ml filtered water
30 drops orange essential oil
20 drops lemongrass essential oil
10 drops neroli essential oil

1. Pour the water and essential oils into a 200 ml spray bottle and shake well.
2. Shake the mixture daily and, after 1 week, decant the mixture and strain it through a muslin cloth.
3. Re-bottle the mixture and shake well before use.

How do I use the room spray? Shake well before use. Spray into the room to refresh the air and to release a fresh citrus aroma throughout your home.

Classic linen spray

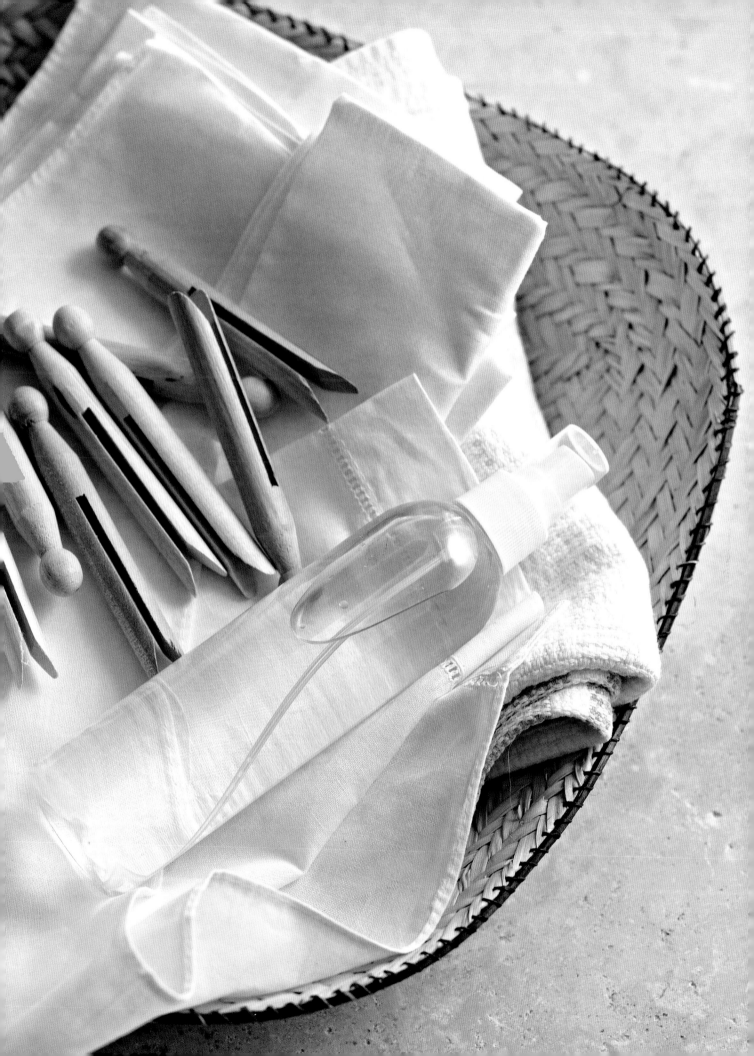

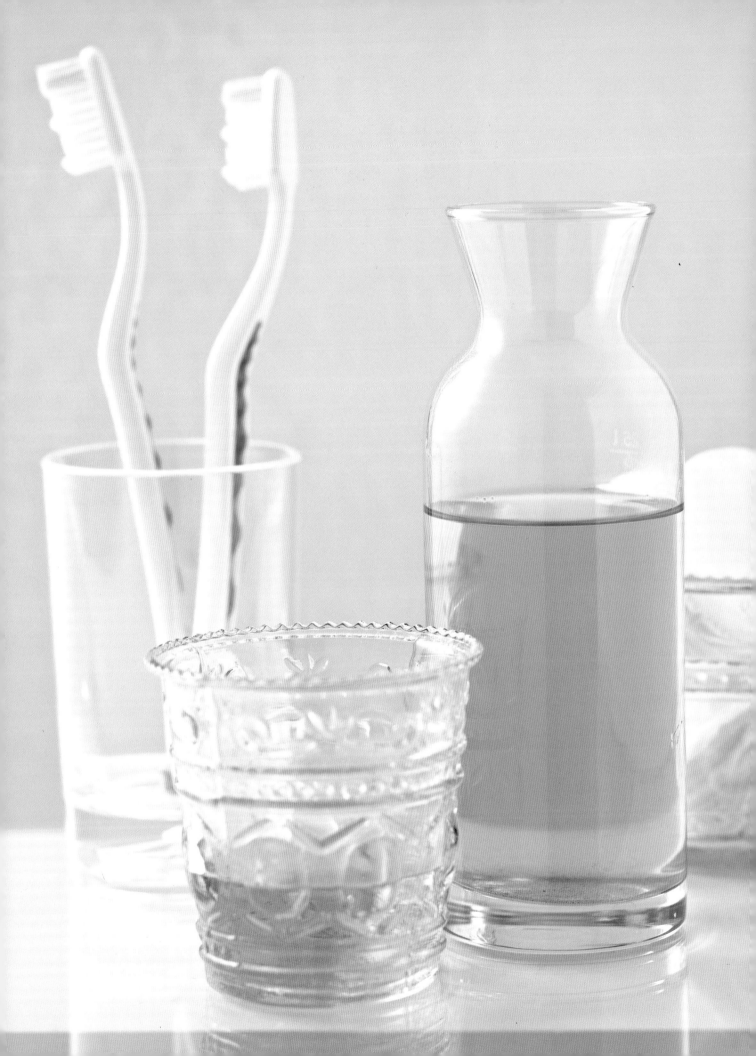

Anti-bacterial and refreshing bathroom air-freshener

200 ml filtered water

20 drops lavender essential oil

20 drops peppermint essential oil

30 drops lemon essential oil

10 drops tea tree essential oil

1. Pour the water and essential oils into a 200 ml spray bottle and shake well.
2. Shake the mixture daily and, after 1 week, decant the mixture and strain it through a muslin cloth.
3. Re-bottle the mixture and shake well before use.

How do I use the air-freshener?
Shake well before use. Spray into the room to refresh the air.

Herbal mouthwash

IT IS NOT RECOMMENDED TO STORE THIS MOUTHWASH FOR LONGER THAN 1 WEEK.

5 ml apple cider vinegar

1 drop peppermint essential oil

250 ml filtered water

1. Place all the ingredients in a glass tumbler and mix well.

How do I use the mouthwash? Stir vigorously before use. Gargle and rinse after brushing your teeth. Do not swallow! Use daily, or as required.

Tip: If you do not enjoy the taste of the apple cider vinegar, substitute with 5 ml vodka.

Herbal mouthwash

Citronella and lemongrass soy candles

CITRONELLA AND LEMONGRASS ESSENTIAL OILS ARE WELL-KNOWN INSECT REPELLANTS – MOSQUITOES
AND FLIES ESPECIALLY DO NOT LIKE THE AROMA OF THESE ESSENTIAL OILS. SOY CANDLE WAX IS DERIVED
FROM THE SOYA BEAN. THE SOY WAX IS EXTREMELY NOURISHING FOR THE SKIN, AND CAN BE USED TO MOISTURIZE
AND TREAT DRY SKIN. ONCE THE CANDLE IS BURNING, AND SOME WAX HAS MELTED, CAREFULLY DIP YOUR FINGER
INTO THE MELTED WAX – BE CAREFUL NOT TO BURN YOUR FINGER ON THE FLAME, AND USE THE LIQUID MELTED WAX
TO RUB INTO THE SKIN. THE BURNING CANDLES WILL ALSO HELP TO REPEL INSECTS IN THE ROOM.

MAKES 3 CANDLES

3 x 15-cm candlewick lengths
   (LX20 thickness)
3 candlewick sustainers
1 pair pliers
silicone glue (available from
   hardware stores)
3 whiskey glass tumblers
500 g soy candle wax
10 ml citronella essential oil
   (1 small bottle)
5 ml lemongrass essential oil
   (½ small bottle)

1. Prepare the glass tumblers the evening before and allow to set overnight.
2. Push the wicks through the candlewick sustainers and squash the centre of the wick sustainer with a pair of pliers to keep the wick in place.
3. Squeeze a small amount of silicone glue onto the bottom of the glass tumblers, in the centre. Press the smooth side of the wick sustainer onto the glue and allow to set overnight.
4. Heat the soy candle wax in a saucepan over low heat until completely melted. Stir in the essential oils.
5. Holding the wicks upright, pour the mixture into the glasses and allow to set.
6. Once the candles have set, trim the wicks using scissors.

Helpful hint: Massage some of the melted candle wax onto the legs and arms as an effective mosquito repellant when camping or sitting outside in the evenings.

Bug away spray

THE ESSENTIAL OILS IN THIS RECIPE ARE KNOWN INSECT REPELLANTS. SPRAY THE AIR, AS WELL AS A LITTLE ON YOUR BODY TO
HELP DETER INSECTS. CITRONELLA OIL IS VERY EFFECTIVE AGAINST MOSQUITOES AND IS OFTEN USED IN CANDLES AND SPRAYS
TO KEEP THEM – AND FLIES – AWAY, THE NATURAL WAY!

MAKES 200 ML

200 ml filtered water
20 drops citronella essential oil
10 drops basil essential oil
10 drops geranium essential oil
10 drops lemongrass essential oil

1. Pour the water and essential oils into a 200 ml spray bottle and shake well.
2. Shake the mixture daily and, after 1 week, decant the mixture and strain it through a muslin cloth.
3. Re-bottle the mixture and shake well before use.

How do I use the bug spray? Shake well before use. Spray into the room to deter mosquitoes and bugs. Spray lightly onto arms and legs to repel mosquitoes.

Citronella and lemongrass soy candles

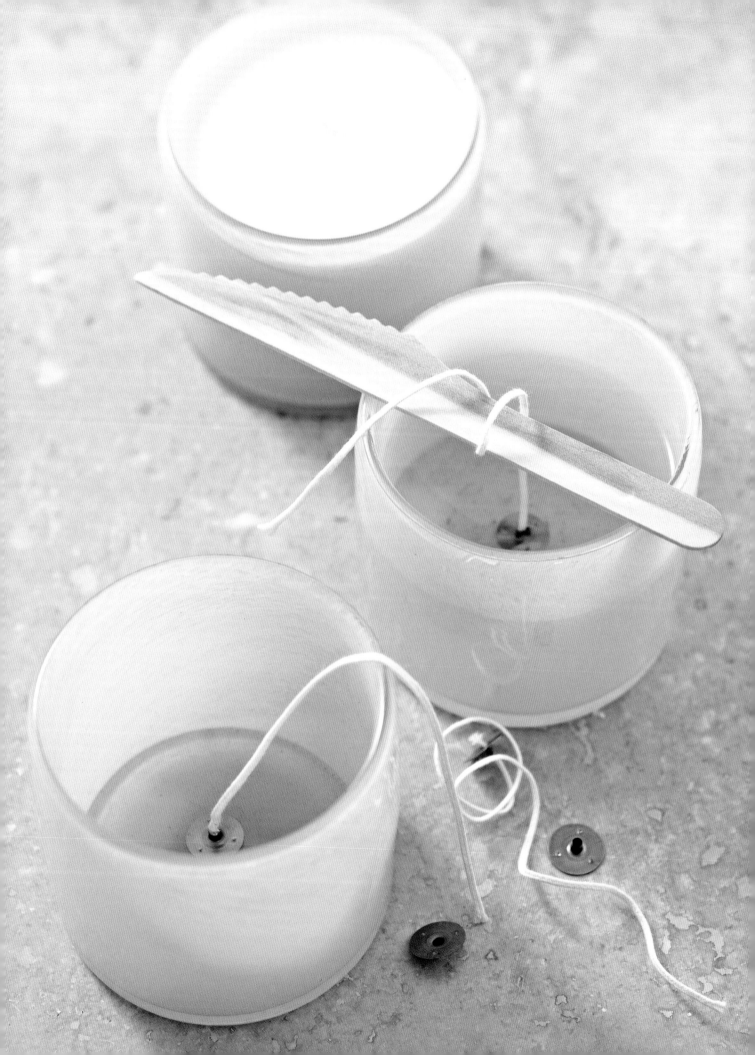

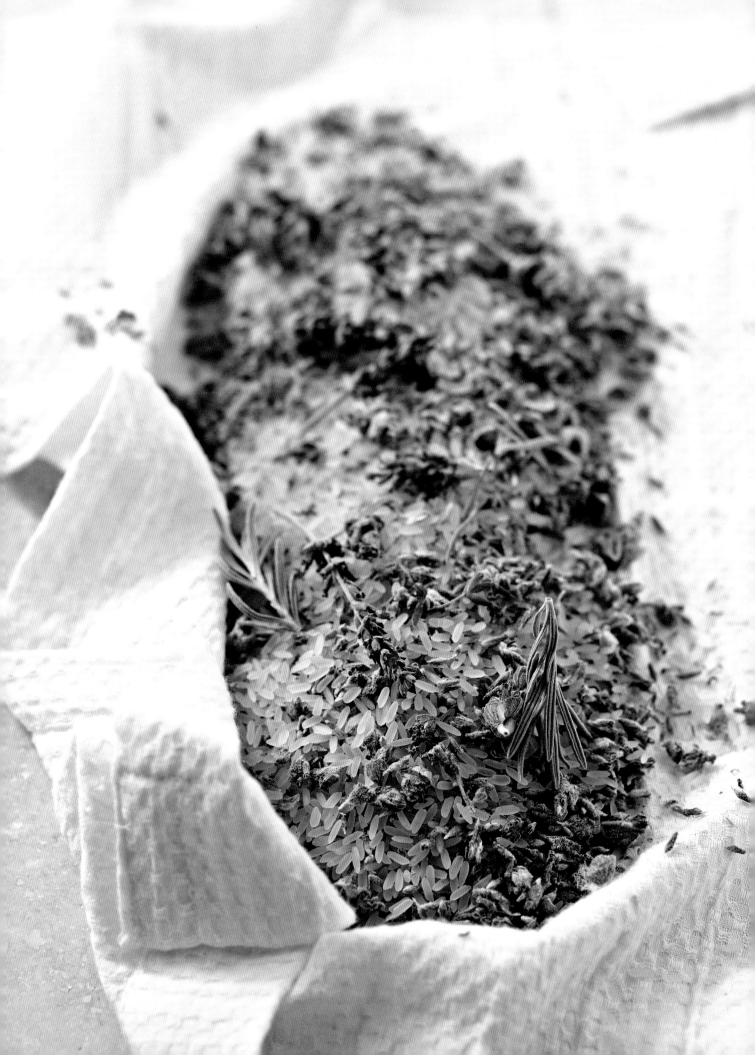

Lavender and rice heat pad

THIS FRAGRANT HEAT PAD WILL SEE YOU THROUGH EVEN THE COLDEST WINTERS! IDEAL TO USE INSTEAD OF A HOT-WATER BOTTLE, THIS HEAT PAD CAN ALSO BE SLUNG OVER YOUR NECK AND SHOULDERS TO RELIEVE TIGHT MUSCLES AND TO EASE MUSCULAR ACHES AND PAINS. IT IS ALSO VERY EFFECTIVE AS A WARMING AND PAIN-RELIEVING TOOL FOR BACKACHE AND PMS.

MAKES 1 HEAT PAD

thick cotton material (or calico) measuring 50 x 25 cm to make the rice bag
250 ml dried lavender flowers
5 x 250 ml raw white rice

1. Fold the material in half lengthways and use a sewing machine to sew along the side and bottom to make the shape of a long tubular bag.
2. Turn the bag inside out so that the seams are on the inside.
3. Break up the lavender flowers and place in a bowl. Add the rice and mix well.
4. Spoon the lavender/rice mixture into the bag. The bag should be about three-quarters full.
5. Turn the open ends inwards and sew the top end of the bag closed.

Helpful hint: Make a drawstring bean bag cover out of muslin or toweling material. The drawstring bean bag cover can be easily washed and dried for hygiene purposes. Heat the lavender heat pad in the microwave before inserting into the drawstring cover.

How do I use the heat pad?

Warm the lavender rice bag (without the protective cover) in the microwave oven for 4 minutes on high or full power. Slip the heated lavender bag into its protective cover.

I use my lavender heat pad a lot in winter for massages (as a heating aid for muscular aches and pains and relaxation), about three times a day. I create a new heat pad every winter.

The outer protective covering (or drawstring bag) should be washed when it starts to get dirty or grubby. You can also wrap the heat pad in some paper towel or tissue if you want to place the heat pad directly onto your skin (and your skin has oil or cream on it). This maintains hygiene and prevents the protective cover from getting dirty too quickly.

Lavender and rice heat pad

First-aid and medicinal products

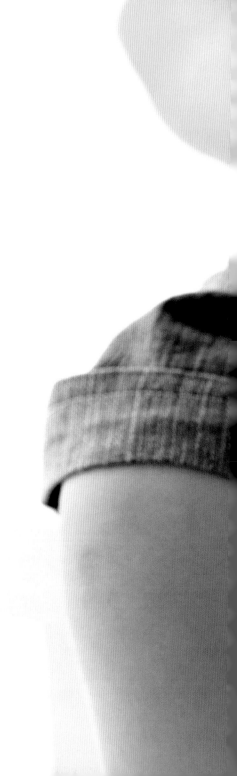

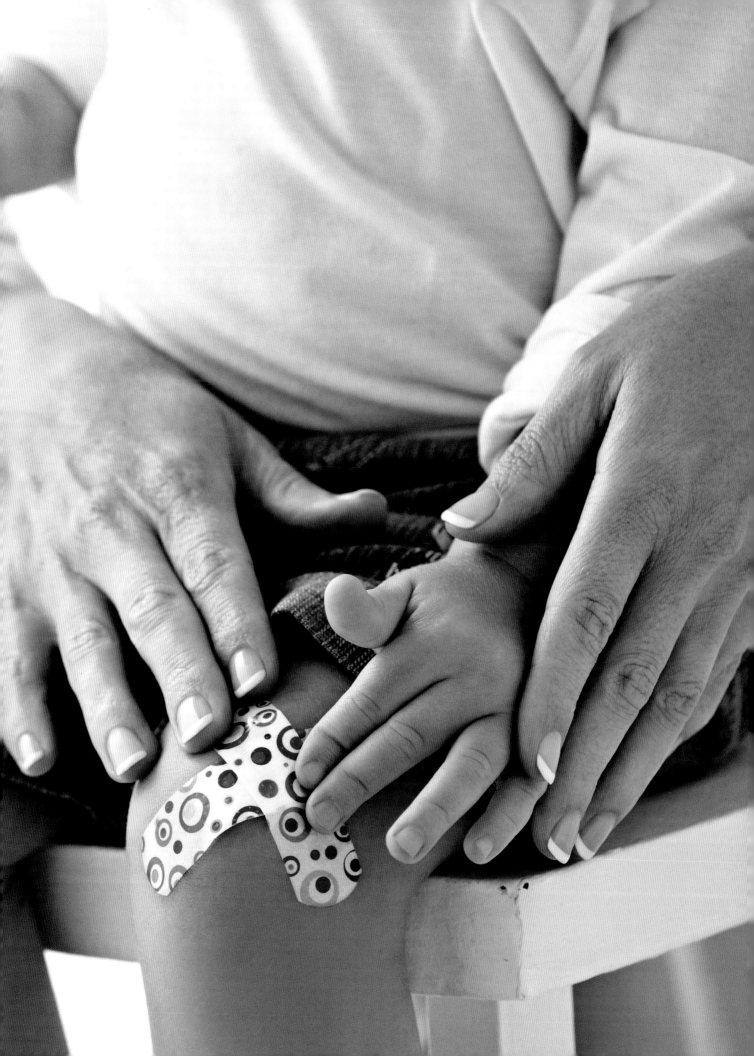

Disinfectant wound cleanser

USE THIS NATURAL WOUND CLEANSER WITH TEA TREE, BERGAMOT AND LAVENDER AROMATHERAPY OILS TO HELP CLEAN AND DISINFECT MINOR WOUNDS, CUTS AND SCRAPES.

MAKES 50 ML

5 ml apple cider vinegar
50 ml distilled or filtered water
2 drops tea tree essential oil
1 drop lavender essential oil
1 drop bergamot essential oil

1. Mix all the ingredients together and pour into a sterilized glass or plastic container. Shake well.

How do I use the wound cleanser? Dip cotton wool into the wound cleanser and cleanse the wound gently. Discard the mixture once you have used it. It is advised to make up a fresh batch for each application.

CAUTION: Do not use on deep wounds, or near the eyes and nose. Not to be used internally.

Mouthwash for sore throats

HONEY IS SOOTHING FOR A SORE THROAT (TRY TO USE RAW HONEY, AS IT HAS NOT BEEN BOILED AND STILL CONTAINS ALL THE NATURAL GOODNESS). SAGE, APPLE CIDER VINEGAR AND TEA TREE ARE USED FOR THEIR ANTI-MICROBIAL PROPERTIES AND MAY HELP TO KEEP A SORE THROAT FROM DEVELOPING INTO A THROAT INFECTION.

MAKES ABOUT 125 ML

handful of sage leaves
125 ml boiling water
5 ml apple cider vinegar
5 ml honey
1 drop tea tree essential oil

1. Prepare a cup of herbal tea with a large handful of fresh sage leaves. Pour the boiling water over the sage leaves and allow the herbal tea to draw for 10 minutes.
2. Measure 125 ml of the tea. Add the apple cider vinegar, honey and essential oil and stir well.
3. Make sure that the mixture is warm – not too hot – before gargling and rinsing the mouth.

How do I use the mouthwash? Gargle frequently with the mouthwash when you have a sore throat, and use up this amount within a day. This mixture will not keep well and so needs to be made daily when required.

Disinfectant wound cleanser

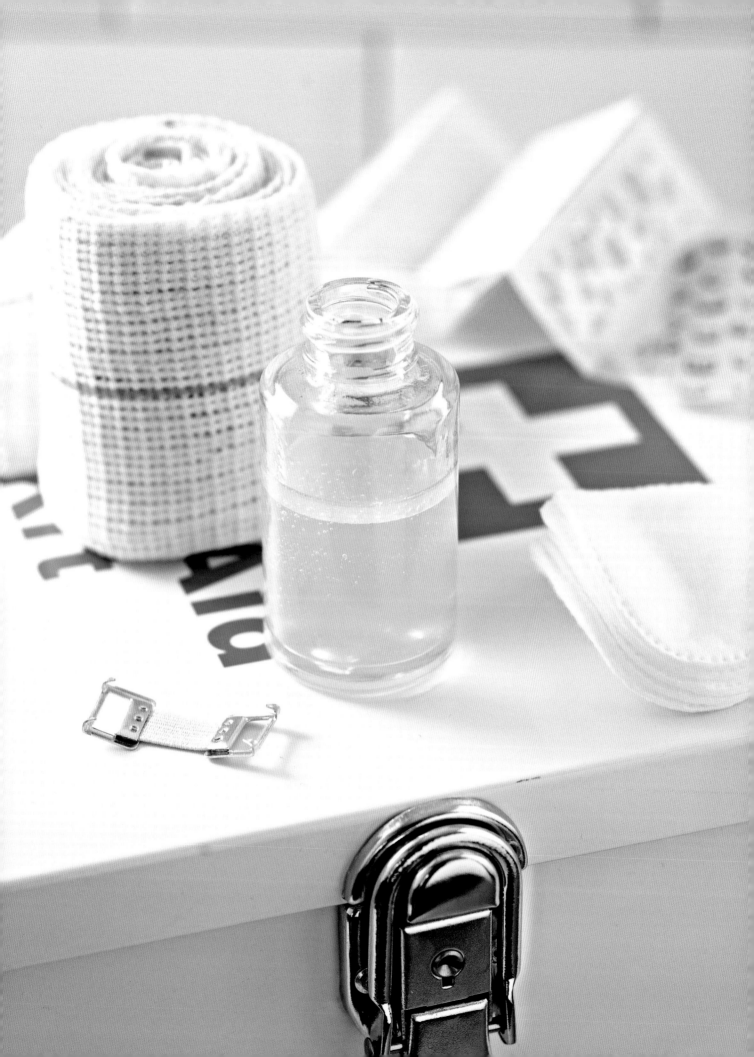

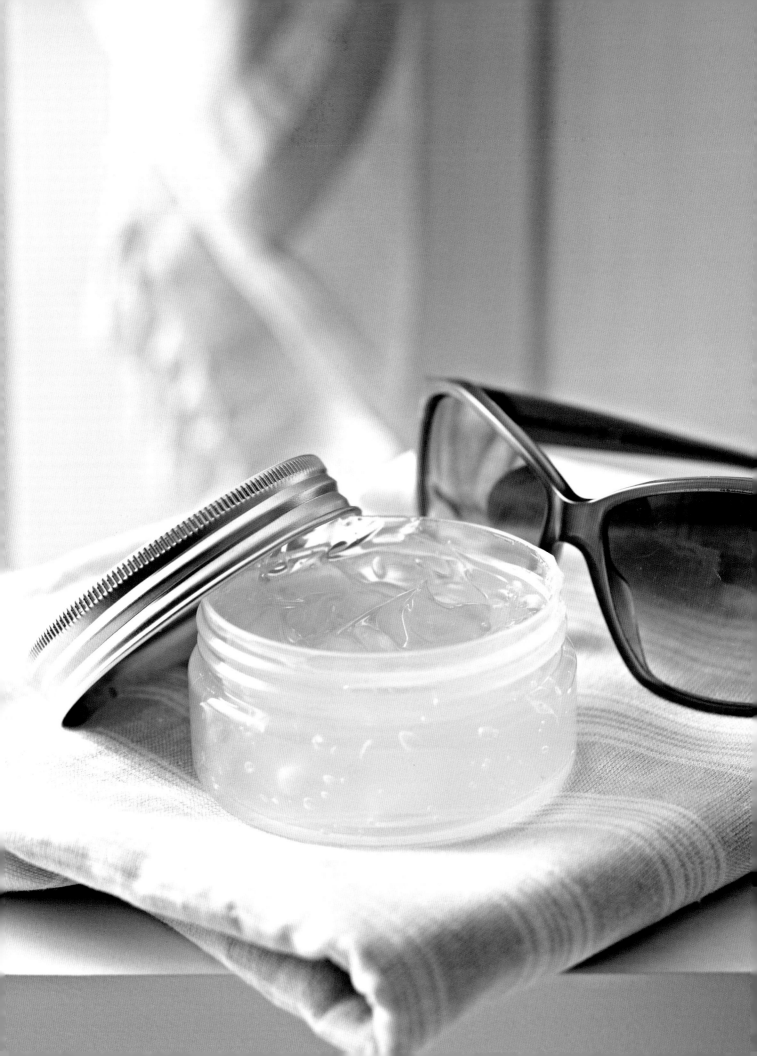

Lavender after-sun gel

MOST PEOPLE USE SUNSCREEN, BUT SUNBURN CAN ALSO OCCUR DUE TO PEOPLE NOT RE-APPLYING SUNSCREEN
AFTER SWIMMING AND TOWEL DRYING. I PREFER TO USE A NATURAL SUNSCREEN PRODUCT THAT DOESN'T CONTAIN CHEMICALS.
SUNUMBRA IS A VERY EFFECTIVE NATURAL SUNSCREEN THAT IS GENTLE ENOUGH TO USE ON EVEN THE MOST SENSITIVE SKIN.
SEE STOCKISTS FOR DETAILS FOR SUNUMBRA SPF 30 AND SPF 40.
THIS AFTER-SUN GEL IS ONE OF MY BEST SELLERS. I STRONGLY RECOMMEND THAT YOU RATHER AVOID SUNBURN,
BUT IF YOU HAVE BEEN CAUGHT OUT, THEN THIS GEL WORKS WONDERS!

MAKES 250 ML

250 ml carrier gel
40 drops lavender essential oil
4 drops peppermint essential oil
4 drops German chamomile essential oil

1. Place the carrier gel in a glass or plastic mixing bowl. Add the essential oils and mix until the oils are fully incorporated into the gel. The gel may turn a slight milky colour due to the high concentration of essential oils but this is normal.
2. Spoon into a sterilized glass or plastic jar.

How do I use the after-sun gel? Apply liberally to sunburned skin.

Tip: Place the gel in the fridge for a few minutes before you apply to sunburned skin. The gel will become very cool and is very soothing.

Spot-control gel for pimples and blemishes

THIS GEL CAN BE APPLIED DIRECTLY TO PIMPLES TO FACILITATE HEALING AND TO TREAT INFLAMMATION. THE TEA TREE AND
LAVENDER ESSENTIAL OILS PREVENT SCARRING AND ARE RENOWNED FOR THEIR ANTI-BACTERIAL AND SOOTHING PROPERTIES.
PROPOLIS EXTRACT (A BROWN RESINOUS SUBSTANCE THAT BEES COLLECT FROM THE LEAVES AND BARK OF POPLAR AND
CONIFER TREES) IS HIGH IN ANTIOXIDANTS AND IS ALSO ANTI-BACTERIAL AND AN EFFECTIVE WOUND HEALER.

MAKES 50 ML

50 ml carrier gel
5 drops propolis extract
15 drops tea tree essential oil
5 drops lavender essential oil

1. Mix the carrier gel and propolis extract together.
2. Add the essential oils and mix well.
3. Spoon into a sterilized glass or plastic jar.

How do I use the gel? Apply a little gel directly to pimples to encourage healing and to ease inflammation.

Lavender after-sun gel

Dry skin relief cream

COMBAT DRY AND ITCHY SKIN WITH THIS HEALING AND SOOTHING CREAM. THE CALENDULA-INFUSED OIL HELPS TO SOOTHE SKIN IRRITATIONS, WHILE THE ESSENTIAL OILS OF LAVENDER, GERMAN CHAMOMILE AND SANDALWOOD ARE WELL KNOWN FOR THEIR CALMING, HEALING AND ANTI-INFLAMMATORY EFFECTS ON THE SKIN. I HAVE RECOMMENDED THIS SOOTHING CREAM FOR MANY CLIENTS WITH ECZEMA AND DERMATITIS. REMEMBER: INFLAMMATORY SKIN CONDITIONS ARE OFTEN A RESULT OF AN UNDERLYING CONDITION AND, IF YOUR SKIN CONDITION DOES NOT IMPROVE, I RECOMMEND A CONSULTATION WITH YOUR LOCAL NATUROPATH/HOMEOPATH TO HELP TO CORRECT THE IMBALANCE WITHIN THE BODY.

MAKES 250 ML

20 ml shea butter
200 ml thickened carrier cream
30 ml calendula-infused oil (see below)
12 drops lavender essential oil
10 drops German chamomile
**   essential oil**
6 drops sandalwood essential oil

1. Heat the shea butter in a small saucepan over very low heat until it has just melted.
2. Place the melted shea butter in the fridge to solidify – this should take about 15 minutes. Remove from the fridge when the shea butter is the consistency of very soft butter.
3. Place the thickened carrier cream in a glass or plastic mixing bowl and add the calendula-infused oil. Mix well.
4. Add the carrier cream/calendula oil mixture to the shea butter and mix well.
5. Stir in the essential oils and spoon into a sterilized glass or plastic jar.

How do I apply the cream? Apply daily to the affected area to help soothe very dry skin conditions. Re-apply after bathing or showering or whenever your skin is very dry.

HOW TO MAKE THE CALENDULA-INFUSED OIL:
Place 50 ml calendula petals and 30 ml sweet almond oil in a heat resistant glass or ceramic bowl suspended over a saucepan of simmering water and heat very gently for 10 minutes. Remove the glass or ceramic bowl (containing the petals and oil) from the heat, and allow the calendula petals to infuse into the sweet almond oil for a further 20 minutes. Strain.

Dry skin relief cream

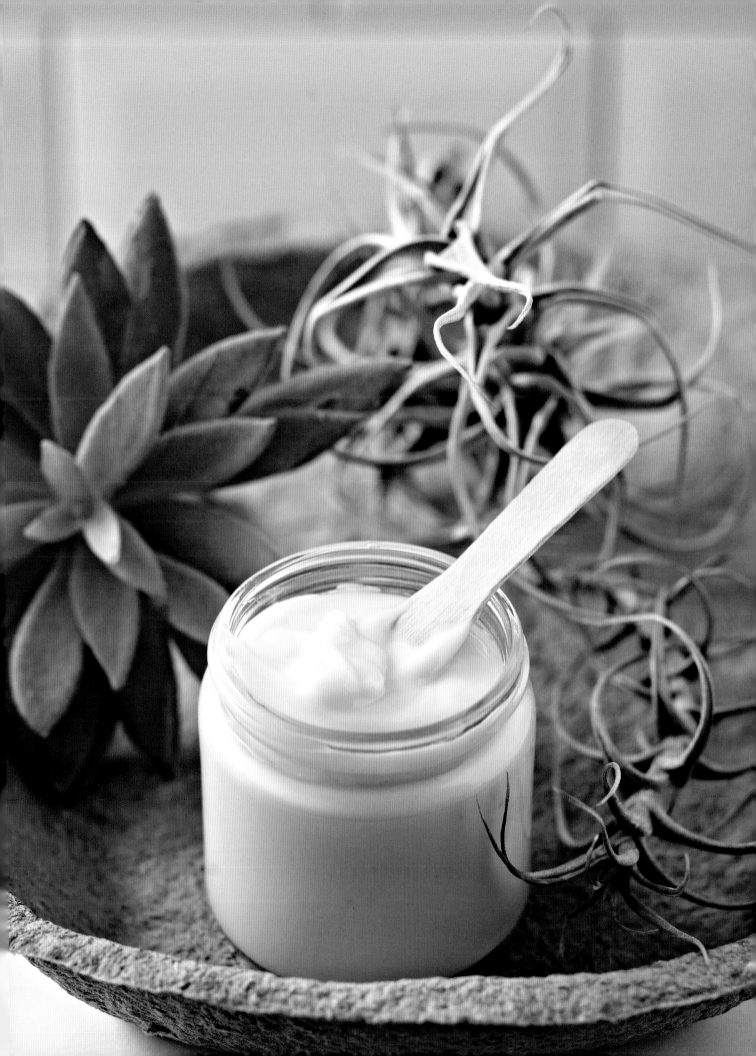

Wrapping and packaging ideas

This is the really fun part of making your own products! This section will show you just how easy it is to decorate your own creations.

RECYCLE OLD GIFT CARDS

I love to recycle old gift cards by simply cutting them to size and punching a hole through one corner. Secure the card to the product with a piece of string or fancy ribbon.

RECYCLE GLASS TUBS (FOR BATH SALTS AND CREAMS)

Re-use your old cosmetic bath salt and cream containers. Remember to wash the containers and sterilize them before filling with your hand-made products.

Add a new label or tag and use decorative wrapping paper, which has been glued with paper glue stick.

Helpful hint: To remove sticky label glue from your glass containers, use neat vinegar. If that doesn't work, try nail-polish remover or pure acetone.

RECYCLE OLD EGG TRAYS

Egg trays make a good container for bath fizz balls – and they also look beautiful when wrapped with cellophane and ribbons.

DIAMANTÉ STICKERS, BEADS AND RIBBONS

Add some 'bling' to your bathroom accessories by gluing nail-art jewels or scrapbook diamanté stickers onto your glass containers. You can find a wide variety of these stickers and ready-made tags and ribbons at your local stationery store.

Attach glass or crystal beads to organza ribbon and tie it around the neck of tall bottles.

CELLOPHANE WRAPPING AND DECORATIVE GIFT WRAPPING PAPER

Aromatherapy soap and fizz balls look great when packaged in clear wrapping, such as cellophane, which shows off their natural textures and colours.

Soap can be packaged in a variety of printed wrapping paper and tied with natural raffia or ribbons.

Use a cellophane packet and decorative ribbons to gift wrap bath salts.

Handy tip: Keep the hard brown cardboard paper (inside the gift wrapping paper roll) and use it to create your own natural brown gift tags. You can also cut decorative wrapping paper and paste it onto the brown cardboard gift tag using paper glue stick. Punch a hole in the top of the tag and fasten to your hand-made product. Only paste wrapping paper on one side if you want to write a note.

DRIED HERBS AND FLOWERS

Dried sprigs of lavender and bay leaves can also be tied onto individual soap bars.

Add rose petals and lavender flowers to clear cellophane when wrapping fizz balls, soap or gift parcels.

GIFT PACKS/HAMPERS/PARCELS

Use clear cellophane as well as colourful printed cardboard bake-in trays (actually used to bake cakes and loaves) to wrap a variety of natural products. These cardboard trays are non-toxic and are recyclable.

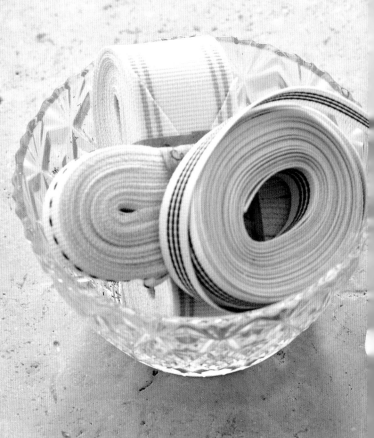

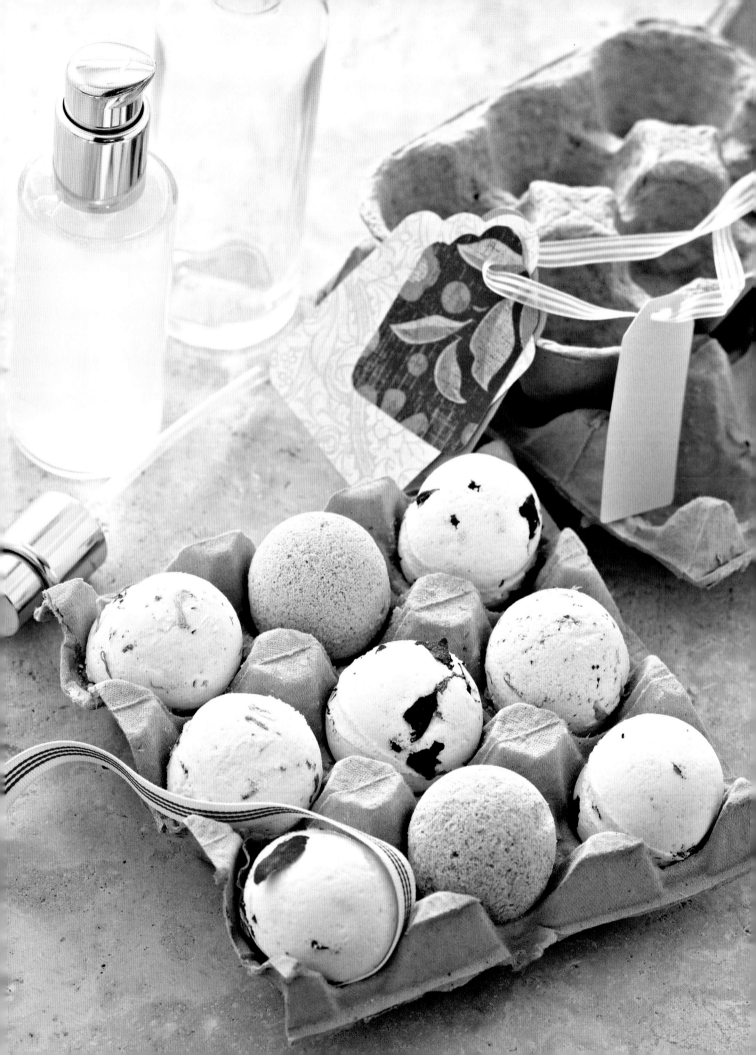

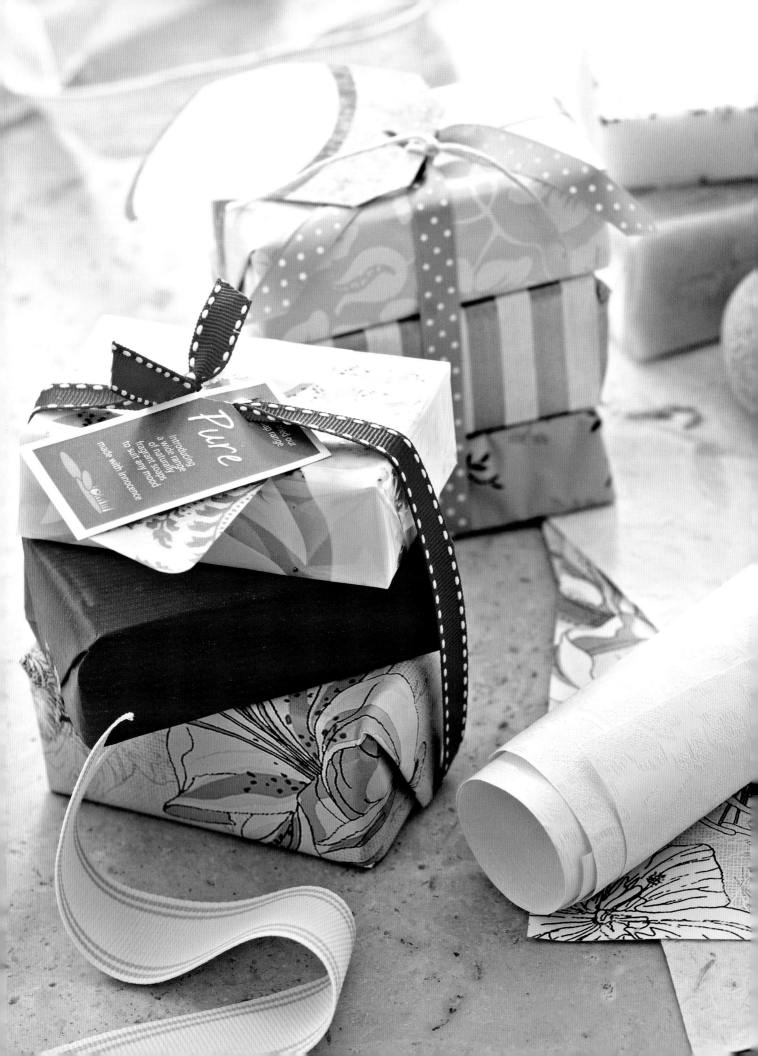

Pure

Introducing
a wide range
of naturally
fragrant soaps
to suit any mood
made with innocence

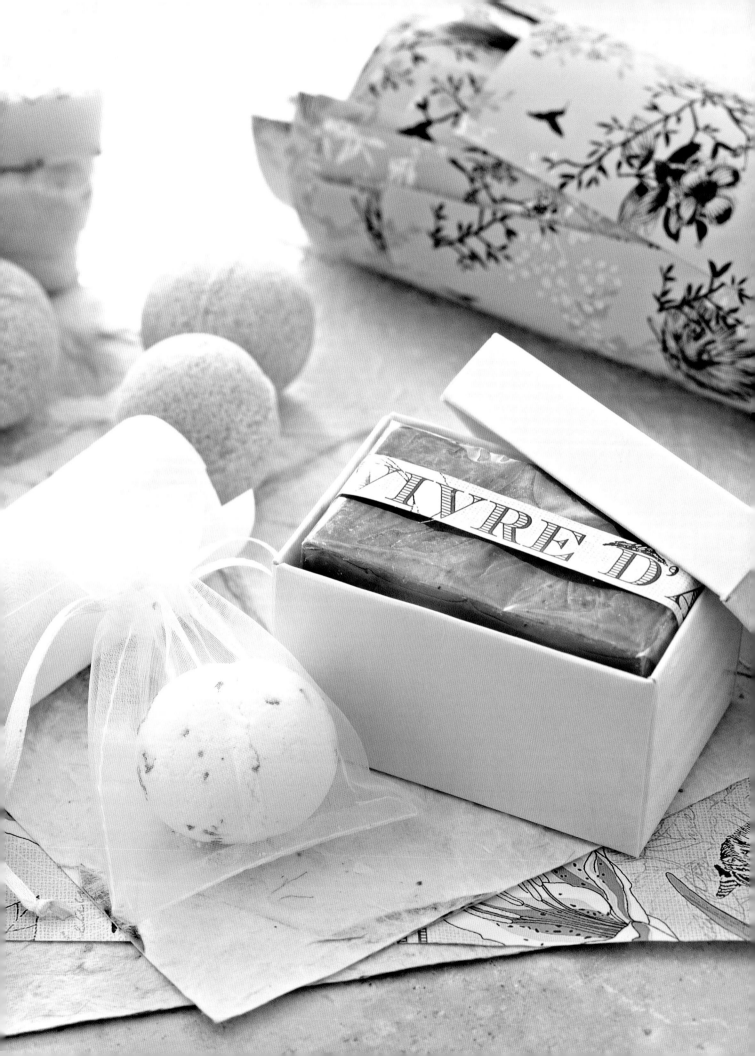

Bibliography

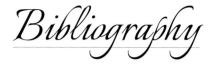

BOOKS

Baser, K.H.C. and Buchbauer, G. 2010. *Handbook of Essential Oils: Science, Technology, and Applications*. CRC Press, Boca Raton, London, New York.

Guide to Aromatherapy. 1995. Geddes & Grosset. ISBN 1-85534-689-3.

Lawless, Julia. 1997. *The Complete Illustrated Guide to Aromatherapy*. Sterling Publishing.

Schnaubelt, Kurt. 1999. *Advanced Aromatherapy: The Science of Essential Oil Therapy*. Healing Arts Press.

Sellar, Wanda. 2001. *The Directory of Essential Oils* (Reprint ed.). Essex: The C.W. Daniel Company, Ltd.

Tisserand, Robert. 1995. *Essential Oil Safety: A Guide for Health Care Professionals*. Churchill Livingstone.

Worwood, Valerie Ann. 1995. *The Fragrant Mind: Aromatherapy for Personality, Mind, Mood and Emotion*. Bantam Books.

WEBSITES

www.makeup2enhance.com
www.cosmeticsinfo.org
www.canserreasearchuk.org
www.preventcancer.com
www.sirc.org
www.slideshare.net
www.alchemy-works.com
www.wikipedia.org
www.herbwisdom.com
www.fromnaturewithlove.com
www.livestrong.com

Stockists and suppliers

Your local supermarket will be able to provide you with the following ingredients:
- Sunflower oil, olive oil (for making soap and aromatherapy products)
- White margarine (for making soap)
- Selected herbal teas (such as rooibos and peppermint), Ceylon tea, Earl Grey tea, as well as ground coffee beans (for adding to soap)
- Rubber gloves (for protecting your hands while making soap)
- Kitchen utensils, such as whisks, spoons, etc.
- Stainless steel saucepans and non-stick pans
- Dishcloths and paper towel
- Sea salt and Himalayan salt
- Bicarbonate of soda and citric acid (for making bath fizz balls)
- Sugar (for body scrub)
- Honey (for soap and scrubs)
- Glass tumblers for candles
- Wrapping paper and gift wrapping tape, ribbons (for wrapping soap and decorating containers and jars)

Your local hardware store will be able to provide you with the following:
- Caustic soda
- Protective plastic sheeting (for protecting work surfaces when making soap and aromatherapy products)
- Protective eye wear (goggles) and dust mask (for wearing while making soap)

Your local health shop will be able to provide you with the following:
- Essential oils
- Carrier oils
- Herbal tea (to add to soap or aromatherapy products)
- Sunumbra SPF 30 and SPF 40

WESTERN CAPE

Candle Maker's Deli
Soap moulds and plain glycerine soap, soy candle wax, candle making equipment, soap thermometers.
46 Marconi Road, Montague Gardens, Cape Town
Tel: (021) 552 4937
Email: sales@candledeli.co.za
Website: www.candledeli.co.za

GB Packaging
Variety of plastic containers for aromatherapy products, as well as amber glass essential oil bottles.
Unit 1, Kiara Square, Esso Road, Montague Gardens, Cape Town
Tel: (021) 551 4374
Email: salesmanager@gbpackaging.co.za
Website: www.gbpackaging.co.za

Honeybee Foundation and Products
Beeswax and honey products.
Tel: (021) 511 4567
Email: honeybee@global.co.za
Website: www.beekeeping.com/honeybee-africa/

Merrypak and Print
Variety of printed giftwrapping paper, paper gift boxes, tissue paper wrapping, cellophane plastic wrapping, printed paper gift bags, raffia, ribbons, beads and general stationery equipment.
45 Morningside Road, Ndabeni, Cape Town
Tel: (021) 531 2244
Website: www.merrypak.co.za

Nature's Way Wellness
Stockists of unfragranced aromatherapy carrier lotions, unfragranced liquid soap, soy candle wax, vegetable-based carrier oils (palm oil, coconut oil, shea butter, cocoa butter), Spalogic essential oils, Saloncare products, dried herbs, rooibos extract, natural soap additives, surfactant-base unfragranced ready-to-use vegetable-based creams, scrubs, lotions, bicarbonate of soda, citric acid, clear and white unfragranced glycerine soap, kaolin clay, Sunumbra SPF 30 and SPF 40.
Beginners and advanced soap making classes and workshops available.
Orders can be couriered anywhere within South Africa.
Tel: (021) 558 6316
Email: nicole@natureswaywellness.co.za
Website: www.natureswaywellness.co.za

Rap Packaging
Variety of plastic containers for aromatherapy products, as well as amber glass essential oil bottles.
Unit F1, Maitland Business Park, 788 Voortrekker Road, Cape Town
Tel: (021) 593 0861
Email: Jennifer@rap.co.za

Saloncare (head office)
Distributors for Cape Town and Gauteng.
Unit 4, Beacon Business Park, Marinus Drive, Montague Gardens, Cape Town
Tel: (021) 552 0216

Serendipity Quintessentials
Dried herbs, alkanet root, annatto seeds, carrier oils, essential oils and aromatherapy hydrosols.
Tel: (021) 531 3545
Email: drsnye@bucknet.co.za

Tocara Skin and Body Science
Stockists of Sunumbra SPF 30 and SPF 40 and Dr. Hauschka products.
Tel: (021) 702 3617
Website: www.tocara4.co.za; www.sunumbra.com

Wellness warehouse
Essential oils, carrier oils (e.g. sweet almond oil, coconut oil, olive oil), dried herbs/herbal tea.
Online store available.
50 Kloof Street, c/o Kloof and Park roads, Cape Town
Tel: 0860 548 3543
Email: community@wellnesswarehouse.com
Website: www.wellnesswarehouse.com

GAUTENG

Fun with Candles
67 Soutpansberg Drive, Kempton Park, Gauteng
Email: debbiecapazorio@gmail.com
Website: www.funwithcandles.co.za

Honeybadger
Stockists of beeswax sheets and beeswax bars and honey.
Plot 239, Kameeldrif, Cnr Moloto and Tambotie streets, Pretoria
Email: anton@honeybadger.co.za
Website: www.honeybadger.co.za

Moco Cosmetic Packaging
Variety of plastic containers for aromatherapy products,
as well as amber glass essential oil bottles.
Orders can be purchased and delivered nationwide via
courier service.
18 Auret Street, Jeppestown, Gauteng
Tel: (011) 624 3493/4
Email: sales@mocopack.co.za
Website: www.mocopackaging.co.za

Packaging Source
Variety of printed wrapping paper, paper gift boxes,
tissue paper wrapping, cellophane plastic wrapping,
printed paper gift bags, raffia, ribbons, beads and
general stationery equipment.
Online store available.
Showroom and shop is located at 54 Hesket drive,
Moreletapark, Pretoria
Tel: (012) 997 0169
Email: sales@packagingsource.co.za
Website: www.packagingsource.co.za

Rap Packaging
Variety of plastic containers for aromatherapy products,
as well as amber glass essential oil bottles.
13 Jersey Drive, Unit 5 Brett Park, Longmeadow East,
Longmeadow Business Park,
Johannesburg
Tel: (011) 590 1598
Email: Sales@rap.co.za
Website: www.rap.co.za

The Flower Spot
Stockists of ribbons, cardboard printed gift boxes and
wrapping paper.
Shop 6, Woodmead Value Mart, Waterval Crescent,
Woodmead, Sandton
Tel: (011) 804 5468
Email: info@flowerspot.co.za
Website: www.flowerspot.co.za

Windrose
Suppliers of essential oils and carrier oils.
Online store available.
Tel: (011) 454 5400
Email: info@windrose.co.za
Website: www.windrose.co.za

EASTERN CAPE

Menno's Bees
Suppliers of honey and hive products.
Honeycombe Farm, Kragga Kamma Road, Theescombe,
Port Elizabeth
Tel: (041) 367 3100
Website: http://mennosbees.com/

Total Concept Distributors
Distributors of Saloncare products.
67–69 Pickering Street, Newton Park
Tel: (041) 365 1472
Email: info@totalconcept.co.za
Website: www.totalconcept.co.za

KWAZULU-NATAL

Ambrosia Apiaries
Suppliers of honey and hive products, including
confectionary and crafts (e.g. beeswax candles), and
honey health-related products (e.g. propolis).
Fig Trees Farm, Inanda Road, Hillcrest
Tel: 083 225 5126

Rap Packaging
Variety of plastic containers for aromatherapy products,
as well as amber glass essential oil bottles.
40 Alexander Road, Westmead
Tel: (031) 700 3595
Email: Zeonie@rap.co.za

SOiL
Certified organic essential oils and carrier oils and
aromatherapy hydrosols.
Online store available.
Tel: (035) 340 7008
Website: www.soil.co.za

Upfront Distributors
Distributors of Saloncare products.
55 Smiso Nkwanyana (Goble Road), Morningside,
Durban
Tel: (031) 312 3502
Email: info@upfrontdistribution.com
Website: www.upfrontdistribution.com

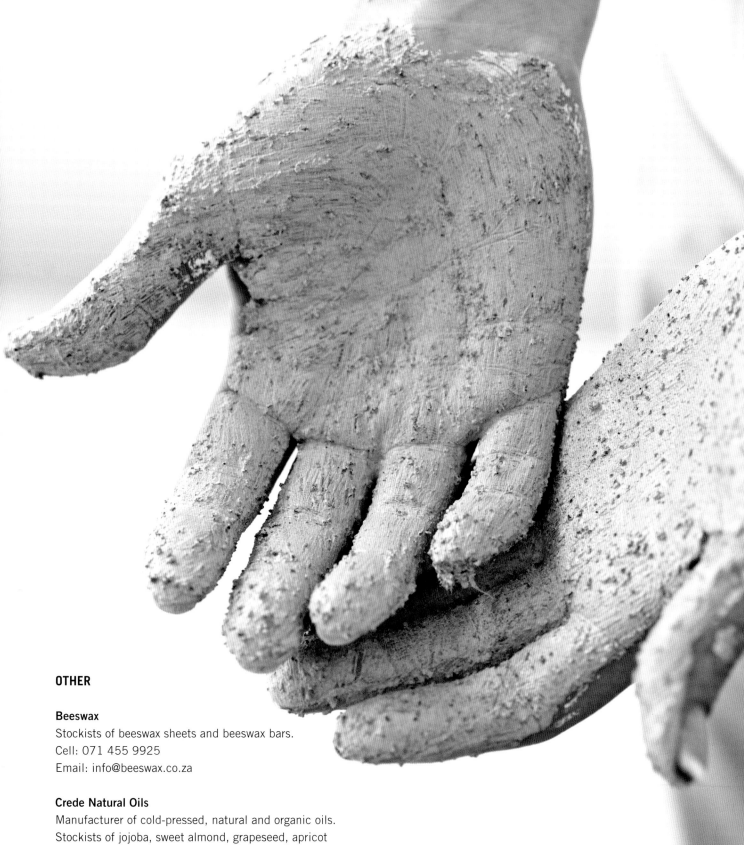

OTHER

Beeswax
Stockists of beeswax sheets and beeswax bars.
Cell: 071 455 9925
Email: info@beeswax.co.za

Crede Natural Oils
Manufacturer of cold-pressed, natural and organic oils.
Stockists of jojoba, sweet almond, grapeseed, apricot
kernels and coconut oils.
Online store available.
Email: info@credeoils.com
Website: www.credeoils.com

Index

Page numbers in **bold** indicate photographs

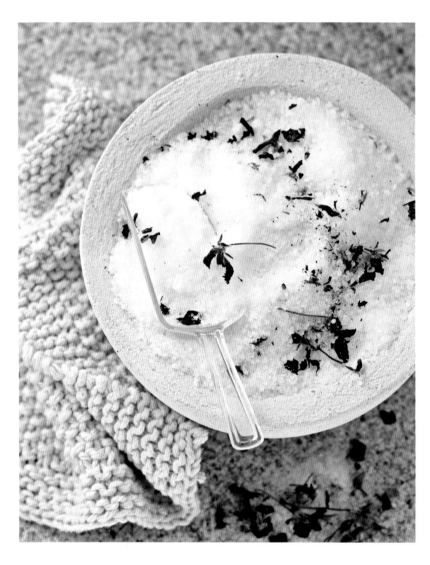

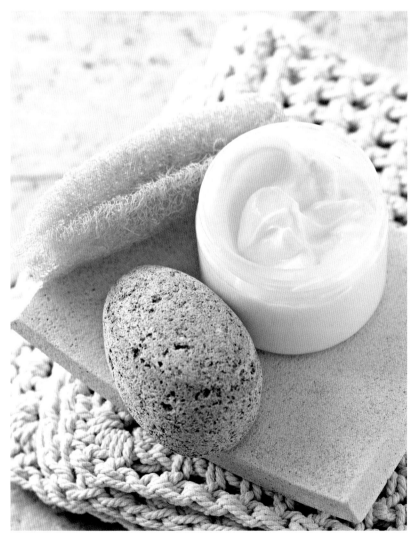

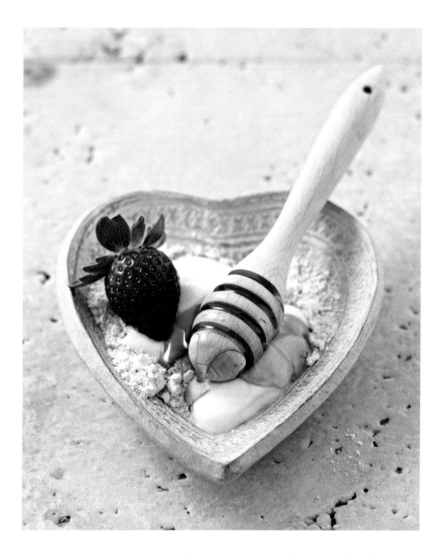

Acknowledgements

To my family – thank you for all your support and encouragement throughout this past year. To my parents, Robbie and Trish Christian, for their unconditional love and care, and my husband, Mark, for assisting me with the QR codes in the book and for your ideas, motivation and suggestions. Most of all, thank you for being such a supportive husband to me, and loving father to our son, Ethan.

I would also like to thank the team behind the book – Linda de Villiers and Steve Connolly from Random House Struik, for giving me the opportunity to publish this book; Joy Clack, for the meticulous editing; Thank you to Bev Dodd and her team for their enthusiasm and creative input, as well as Brita du Plessis and Vaune Desmarais for the styling of this book; and Warren Heath and Mike Levenson for the stunning photographs.

Thank you to everyone who has inspired me to write this book, and a very special thanks to my friends and clients for your suggestions and feedback on my products and recipes.

Happy soap making everyone!

NICOLE SEABROOK

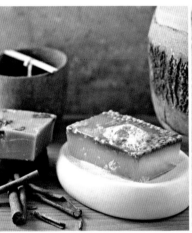 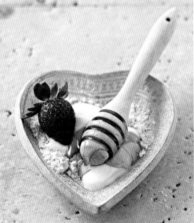 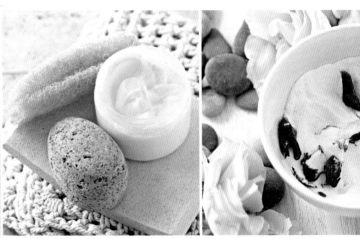

Published in 2013 by Struik Lifestyle
an imprint of Random House Struik (Pty) Ltd
Company Reg. No 1966/003153/07
Wembley Square, 1st Floor, Solan Street, Gardens 8001
PO Box 1144, Cape Town 8000

Visit **www.randomstruik.co.za** and subscribe to our newsletter for monthly updates and news.

Copyright © in published edition:
Random House Struik (Pty) Ltd 2013
Copyright © in text: Nicole Seabrook 2013
Copyright © in photographs:
Random House Struik (Pty) Ltd 2013

ISBN 978 1 43230 200 9

Publisher: Linda de Villiers
Managing editor: Cecilia Barfield
Editor and Indexer: Joy Clack
Designer: Beverley Dodd
Photographer: Warren Heath
Photographer's assistant: Mike Leveson
Stylist: Brita du Plessis
Stylist's assistant: Vaune Desmarais
Proofreader: Samantha Fick

Reproduction by Hirt & Carter Cape (Pty) Ltd
Printed and bound by 1010 Printing International Ltd, China

DISCLAIMER
If you are pregnant or have any serious health condition, consult your aromatherapist before using any essential oils. While the author and publisher have made every effort to ensure that the information contained in this book was accurate at the time of going to press, they accept no responsibility for any loss, injury or inconvenience sustained by any person using this book or following the advice given in it.